Women's Edge
HEALTH ENHANCEMENT GUIDE™

Herbs That Heal

Natural Medicine at Its Best

By Arden Moore, Bridget Doherty, and the Editors of

Rodale Press, Inc.
Emmaus, Pennsylvania

Copyright © 1999 by Rodale Press, Inc.
Illustrations copyright © 1999 by Shawn Banner, Laura Stutzman, and Tom Ward

Prevention Health Books for Women and Women's Edge Health Enhancement Guide are trademarks of Rodale Press, Inc.

Printed in the United States of America on acid-free ∞, recycled paper ♻

Library of Congress Cataloging-in-Publication Data

Moore, Arden.
    Herbs that heal : natural medicine at its best / by Arden Moore, Bridget Doherty, and the editors of Prevention Health Books for Women.
        p.   cm. — (Women's edge health enhancement guide)
    Includes index.
    ISBN 1–57954–119–4 hardcover
    1. Herbs—Therapeutic use.   2. Women—Health and hygiene.
I. Doherty, Bridget.   II. Prevention Health Books for Women.
III. Title.   IV. Series.
RM666.H33M654   1999
615'.321'082—dc21   99–28951

Distributed to the book trade by St. Martin's Press

2 4 6 8 10 9 7 5 3 1   hardcover

Visit us on the Web at www.rodalebooks.com, or call us toll-free at (800) 848-4735.

OUR PURPOSE

We inspire and enable people to improve their lives and the world around them.

Herbs That Heal Staff

EDITOR: E. A. Tremblay
STAFF WRITERS: Arden Moore, Bridget Doherty
CONTRIBUTING WRITERS: Deanna Moyer, Nanci Kulig, Sarí Harrar, Sara Altshul O'Donnell
ART DIRECTOR: Darlene Schneck
SERIES ART DIRECTOR: Diane Ness Shaw
SERIES DESIGNER: Lynn N. Gano
COVER AND BOOK DESIGNER: Diane Ness Shaw
ILLUSTRATORS: Shawn Banner, Diane Ness Shaw, Laura Stutzman, Tom Ward
ASSOCIATE RESEARCH MANAGER: Anita C. Small
LEAD RESEARCHERS: Carol J. Gilmore, Shea Zukowski
EDITORIAL RESEARCHERS: Molly Donaldson Brown, Lori Davis, Grete Haentjens, Jennifer L. Kaas, Mary Kittel, Mary S. Mesaros, Kathryn Piff, Elizabeth Shimer
SENIOR COPY EDITORS: Amy K. Kovalski, Karen Neely
LAYOUT DESIGNER: Donna G. Rossi
ASSOCIATE STUDIO MANAGER: Thomas P. Aczel
MANUFACTURING COORDINATORS: Brenda Miller, Jodi Schaffer, Patrick T. Smith

Rodale Healthy Living Books

VICE PRESIDENT AND PUBLISHER: Brian Carnahan
VICE PRESIDENT AND EDITORIAL DIRECTOR: Debora T. Yost
VICE PRESIDENT AND MARKETING DIRECTOR: Karen Arbegast
EDITORIAL DIRECTOR: Michael Ward
WRITING DIRECTOR: Brian Paul Kaufman
PRODUCT MARKETING MANAGER: Guy Maake
BOOK MANUFACTURING DIRECTOR: Helen Clogston
MANUFACTURING MANAGERS: Eileen Bauder, Mark Krahforst
RESEARCH MANAGER: Ann Gossy Yermish
COPY MANAGER: Lisa D. Andruscavage
PRODUCTION MANAGER: Robert V. Anderson Jr.
OFFICE MANAGER: Jacqueline Dornblaser
OFFICE STAFF: Julie Kehs, Suzanne Lynch, Mary Lou Stephen, Catherine E. Strouse

Prevention Health Books for Women Board of Advisors

The Herbal Alternative

There has been a revolution in self-healing, and women have led it.

It began in backyard gardens, porch planters, windowsill boxes. It mixed the magical with the practical, poetry with medicine. Its lifeblood was lore handed down by grandmothers and great-grandmothers. And its heart was growth and soil.

You've heard plenty about it: the herbal revolution. But what you may not have heard is that it offers lots of satisfactions beyond healing. Herbs can also relax us, stimulate us, and add taste, scent, color, and texture to our lives.

This book is your tour guide to that world. You'll learn how to use herbs medicinally for dozens of common conditions, among them dock root for anemia, guggul for high cholesterol, and nettle for muscle cramps. You'll even discover which herbs can help you quit smoking.

You'll also find out how to use a sprig of basil to pass a test, mugwort to have pleasant dreams, and apple to look younger. You'll ward off envy with rue, and you'll relax with herbal massage oils as well as learn which herbs to use for symptoms of PMS, perimenopause, and menopause.

As with every book in the Women's Edge series, *Herbs That Heal* will give you practical ideas for maintaining your health, youth, and joy in living, in addition to hundreds of specific uses for herbs.

Every new journey has its cautions, of course, and so does this one: When using herbs medicinally, never combine them with prescription drugs unless you check with your doctor first. Likewise, herbs alone can't treat serious or chronic illnesses. And don't use herbs if you're pregnant or nursing unless a medical doctor gives you the okay. In general, use them in combination with a healthy lifestyle, professional medical care, and the counsel of an herbal expert when you need it.

Remember also that herbs, like all medicinal remedies, can have side effects, so please read the precautions in the Safe Use of Herbs and Essential Oils charts at the back of this book before treating yourself.

Now let's get to the fun part: Good reading and good health!

Debora T. Yost

Debora T. Yost
Editorial Director

Contents

PART ONE
The New Age of Herbs

They're Back! Herbs as
Modern-Day Healers **2**

Picking and Choosing
Made Easy **7**

Feel-Good Therapies **16**

PART TWO
Herbal Know-How

50 Herbs Every Woman
Should Know. **30**

PART THREE
Herbs for Body and Soul

The Serenity Herbs **58**

The Energizing Herbs **63**

Smart Healing with Herbs **67**

Safe Use of Herbs
in This Book. **167**

Safe Use of Essential Oils
in This Book. **171**

Herb Index **173**

Subject Index. **176**

The New Age of Herbs

They're Back! Herbs as Modern-Day Healers

Suddenly, herbs are everywhere you look. In health food stores, drugstores, and even supermarkets, echinacea sits next to cold and flu decongestants. Plants with names so magical they sound perfect for casting spells, such as ginkgo and black cohosh, line the shelves. You'd think we were witnessing a breakthrough in modern medicine. But these "modern" remedies have healed people for thousands and thousands of years.

Herbs were used to cure ills ranging from aches and pains and menstrual problems to insomnia and depression centuries before modern medicine invented drugs. Here are just a few ways in which herbs have helped to heal people throughout the ages.

- The women of ancient Greece drank wine in which chasteberry leaves had been steeped to regulate their menstrual cycles.
- Garlic, which doctors acknowledge has cholesterol-reducing powers, dates back at least 5,000 years as a healing gem.
- People in ancient Africa applied the gel from the aloe plant to wounds from poisoned arrows, and people of India utilized it as a cooling agent.

- Herbalists 2,000 years ago recommended using ginseng to enlighten the mind and brighten the eyes. Current herbalists prescribe the herb as a tonic that enhances mental function.
- Native Americans took echinacea to treat snakebites, fevers, and stubborn wounds. Early American settlers adopted the plant as a home remedy for colds and flu.
- Soldiers in the Trojan wars treated their wounds with yarrow—a plant used today for cuts and scrapes.

Since the dawn of time, our ancestors depended on plants to nourish them and keep them well. Then, about a hundred years ago, people decided it was time for a change. We turned our backs on our ancient relationship with herbs and looked elsewhere for our food and medicine.

Now, like prodigal children, we're returning to them—in huge numbers. More than 30 percent of the U.S. population relies on herbal alternatives to medically approved drugs. In just a two-year period, sales of echinacea jumped 72 percent, while sales of the depression-fighter

St. John's wort skyrocketed 1,900 percent.

Not only do we have a plethora of herbs to choose from but we also have items of which the herbal healers of yesteryear could never have dreamed: St. John's wort lipstick, essential oil chewing gum, herb-laden workout energy bars. Companies now sponsor major ad campaigns to promote the sale of herbs. Behind this revival are millions of women, just like yourself, who are looking to herbs as a natural source of healing and comfort.

Women and Herbs: A Natural Connection

Herbalism is and always has been honored as a woman's art. Since ancient times, mothers, wives, and daughters have acted as the guardians and gatekeepers of their families' nutrition and health. Men may have brought home the bacon, but women provided the botanicals. Traditionally, women were always the midwives, the health providers, and the herb collectors, says Feather Jones, a professional member of the American Herbalists Guild (AHG) and director of the Rocky Mountain School of Botanical Studies in Boulder, Colorado.

Often through trial and error, the early herbalists began to understand Mother Nature's products and their healing powers. Using intuition, experience, and common sense, these women made good use of the plants

HOW TO MAKE A "GREEN" FIRST-AID KIT

Daily life is peppered with minor medical annoyances like cuts, scrapes, and digestive distresses. Fortunately, herbs help treat them and provide you with fast, effective relief. A variety of medicinal plants act as wound healers, infection fighters, and antiseptics.

Here is what you'll need to put together your very own herbal remedies kit, as recommended by Claudia Cooke, M.D., a holistic doctor in New York City.

❏ Aloe. Apply the gel from inside the plant to minor burns, sunburn, and rashes. At home, keep a plant on a sunny windowsill. For travel, carry a tube of aloe gel.

❏ Goldenseal powder in capsules. Open a capsule and sprinkle the contents onto an infected cut.

❏ Echinacea tincture. Good for treating colds, flu, and infections. For infections, dilute the echinacea in an equal amount of water and apply to the affected area.

❏ Tea tree essential oil. Dilute the tea tree oil with vegetable oil to fight fungal and bacterial infections in cuts, abrasions, and athlete's foot.

❏ Witch hazel tincture. Protects broken skin from infection. Cleans wounds and aids healing of rashes and minor burns.

❏ Arnica. To ease the pain, swelling, and discoloration of bruises, spread on arnica gel. Don't use on broken skin.

❏ Dried calendula flowers. An effective wash for cuts and scrapes. Make a freshly brewed strong tea with one tablespoon petals per cup of boiling water, steep for 20 minutes, strain, and cool. Then use it to wash the cut.

❏ Dried chamomile flowers. Chamomile tea eases digestive discomfort, calms anxiety, and relieves mild insomnia. For eye infections such as pinkeye, strain the flowers from a freshly brewed tea through a coffee filter and allow the tea to cool. Then use it as a wash.

❏ Gingerroot or capsules. For nausea or motion sickness, take ginger as a tea or in capsules or chew it in its crystallized form.

that the earth gave them. "If someone has a burn, you are going to look around and choose a plant that is succulent and juicy—like aloe," says Ginger Webb, the herbal education coordinator for the American Botanical Council in Austin, Texas.

These wise women passed on their herbal knowledge to their daughters and granddaughters, who then added their own experiences to it, eventually creating what we know—and sometimes disregard—as folklore. Folklore ensures that important information filters down to future generations by weaving instructions into a good story—something easy to remember and interesting enough to tell over and over again.

The craft of healing with herbs flourished until the late nineteenth century. The Industrial Revolution and new technology gave birth to the idea that anything nature can do, man can do better. Where the earth gave us meadowsweet and willow bark as pain relievers, science gave us a much stronger medicine in aspirin.

Then came the discovery of penicillin, which lead some to believe that a "magic bullet," a manmade miracle medicine, could cure all our ills, says Ellen Evert Hopman, a professional member of AHG and author of *Tree Medicine, Tree Magic*. People, especially women, started to turn away from herbs.

Naturally, after a few generations passed, a good deal of herbal history was lost. But now, after nearly a half-century of our overusing penicillin and other antibiotics, bacteria are developing immunities to these drugs. Many diseases and infections are becoming harder to cure, says Hopman.

REAL-LIFE SCENARIO
Her "Secret" Has Him on Edge

Annemarie's purse is practically a medicine cabinet with leather straps. At age 46, she was popping pills all day long—a prescription drug for high blood pressure and lots of over-the-counter medicine to ease the hip pain and achy joints of arthritis. At one point, she was taking up to eight pain pills per day, and they were making her stomach terribly upset. Unhappy with taking so many drugs and dealing with their side effects, Annemarie consulted an herbalist who put her on a "secret formula." The herbalist used a lot of unfamiliar words like *adaptogen* and *tonify* to explain how the herbs worked. Now Annemarie isn't really sure what she's taking or why, but she feels so much better that she's thinking of giving up on her medications. This is alarming her husband, who feels she has fallen victim to a quack. Has she?

Quack or not, Annemarie's herbalist isn't doing her any favors by keeping her in the dark. For her own safety, Annemarie needs to know exactly which herbs she's taking and why. While herbal remedies are generally safe and have few side effects, some could cause adverse reactions if she has allergies or is taking prescription drugs.

If her herbalist won't reveal the so-called secret formula, then Annemarie needs to find another herbalist. This time she should check the person's credentials before taking any advice. She could start by asking a few questions: How long

---

Coming Full Circle

Now, after a century of exile, many women find themselves returning to the herbal ways of their ancestors, Jones says.

Why are we seeking solace in herbs again? The reasons are as numerous as the herbs themselves, but here are few of the major ones.

A feeling of empowerment. Many of us have been educated to believe we must hand over our health to another person—specifically, a doctor. But herbalism allows us to take charge of our has she been in practice? Is she a member of any reputable professional organizations such as the American Association of Naturopathic Physicians, the American Herbalists Guild, or the National Institute of Medical Herbalism? Does she have a degree or any kind of training? Naturopathic doctors (N.D.'s), for example, are often trained in the use of herbs. So are some holistic medical doctors and doctors of Oriental medicine. Finally, where did she study? Only three schools—Bastyr University, National College of Naturopathic Medicine, and Southwest College of Naturopathic Medicine and Health Sciences—currently offer accredited programs in naturopathic medicine.

Whether or not Annemarie switches herbalists, she needs to see her regular doctor. Even if she's pain-free and feeling like she's 20 again, she shouldn't take herself off blood pressure medication without talking to her doctor first. While she may feel great, her blood pressure could still be high.

Just feeling better isn't enough. Annemarie also needs to have her questions answered, and she needs to feel comfortable with the person who's giving her health advice.

Expert consulted
Jesse Lynn Hanley, M.D.
Holistic doctor and medical director
Malibu Health and Rehabilitation Center
Malibu, California

own well-being. We can use herbs to stay healthy and prevent sickness. We can even use plant medicines to treat illnesses. "It is very empowering to realize that you can depend on yourself and take care of yourself and your family with herbs," Hopman says.

Further, herbal medicine sometimes has advantages over conventional: In some cases, you can treat what mainstream science cannot. "Conventional medicine falls short when it comes to treating chronic conditions and everyday illnesses like cold and flu. People with those problems are increasingly taking care of themselves with herbs," notes Hopman.

Getting back to nature. In a high-tech world where computers are far more common than gardens, some women feel cut off from their life source. They don't spend as much time with plants, flowers, and wildlife as they would like. Using herbs reconnects them with nature. "It returns a part of yourself back to the earth," Jones says.

Herbalism gives us a new sense of intimacy with the plant world around us. "The more you learn about herbalism, the more amazing it becomes. You learn that a flower growing along the side of the road is a medicinal plant. And that the weeds growing in between your spinach and your tomatoes are medicinal plants. It's consciousness raising," Webb says.

Herbalism connects us with our environment in another way. Because both women and plants are part of the natural world, our bodies instinctively know what to do with herbs. "You are giving your body something that is a known entity. We have evolved with plants, so our bodies know how to read an herb as opposed to a pharmaceutical," Webb says.

A need for gentle and affordable care. When scientists started creating more potent, synthetic versions of herbs in the early part of the twentieth century, people didn't foresee side effects and the fallout of their use, Jones says. Afraid of the overpowering action of pharmaceuticals, women want the milder, yet just as effective, option of herbs.

On a practical level, herbs sometimes offer refuge from the expensive and tangled world of conventional health care. Trips to doctors, spe-

HERBAL KNOWLEDGE QUIZ

Learning about herbs and their special traits can be tricky and confusing. Have fun with this quiz and see what you already know.

1. I can help to jog your memory. I'm also the herb entwined in a bride's bouquet to encourage fidelity between newlyweds.
    A. Forget-me-nots
    B. Fidelity forever
    C. Rosemary

2. In ancient Greece, my name meant "bees." Even today, beekeepers rub my leaves on new hives to entice bees into them.
    A. Stinging nettle
    B. Honeybuns
    C. Lemon balm

3. You curse my appearance in your manicured lawns but enjoy munching on my leaves in a salad. My roasted roots also make an excellent caffeine-free coffee.
    A. Colombian crabgrass
    B. Burning bush
    C. Dandelion

4. Set my schedule by birds, especially swallows. I flower when they arrive and fade when they depart for the season. The irritating orange juice from my stem can get rid of warts and corns.
    A. Happy bird day
    B. Mistle toad
    C. Celandine

5. I'm not pulling your leg, I was actually named after that weak-heeled Greek hero, Achilles. During the Civil War, my powdered leaves helped stop bleeding on wounded Rebel and Union soldiers.
    A. Blue-and-gray heel
    B. Trojan styptic
    C. Yarrow (*Achillea millefolium*)

6. I'm a bit tricky to eat. American colonists used to cook my berries and make tasty preserves. But better not eat fresh-picked berries off my vines—they're poisonous!
    A. George washingberries
    B. Colonial catastrophe
    C. Cramp bark

7. Look closely at my leaf pattern, and you'll see where the design for the club suit in playing cards originated. Before that, I was used as a poison antidote in ancient Greece. My name means "to set free."
    A. Poker face
    B. Liberation clover
    C. Rue

If you answered "C" to all seven questions, count yourself a perfect score. Congratulations!

cialists, and pharmacies all add up financially. In some cases, herbs help offset those costs. "People are tired of side effects; they are tired of the expense of going to the doctor and getting a prescription," Jones notes.

Whatever the reason, self-care with herbal medicine is a powerful experience for many women. For some, it evolves into a way of life, not just a way of healing. "If you start taking tinctures and teas, your lifestyle changes. You don't just take a pill. You help make your medicine. For instance, herbal teas have this wonderful aroma. You slow down to boil the water and steep the plant. You start experiencing your medicine in a different way. You are part of it," Webb says.

Picking and Choosing Made Easy

We are masters of the supermarket. We know how to shop smart, compare prices, and scrutinize food labels. We clip coupons and buy in bulk. We steer clear of sugar-loaded cereals for our children, and we know the real skinny on fat-free chocolate-chip cookies: They're full of hidden calories.

We can be just as masterful at shopping for herbal remedies.

There's no need to feel overwhelmed and confused by a store shelf stocked with a dozen brands of echinacea. Strange-sounding herbs, such as dong quai or skullcap, need not daunt you. Remember, as a shopper, you already have extraordinary skills. Bring them along when you're choosing your herbal products, whether in a health food store, a discount drugstore, a mail-order catalog, a supermarket, a local gym, or the Internet.

Begin at the Beginning

When you buy groceries, you don't usually select items off the shelf on impulse. First you make a shopping list. You determine what ingre-dients you need to make your family's favorite lasagna or apple crisp. You check to see if your bathrooms are low in tissue or toothpaste. You ask your beagle if she needs more dog biscuits (that tail wagging is a dead giveaway).

By the same token, you shouldn't randomly select a handful of medicinal herbs without knowing what their benefits are and how well they match your needs. Herbs can play a vital role in improving and maintaining your health if you choose and plan wisely. Do some research before you shop. Then make a list. Here are some guidelines from herbal practitioners to help you.

Understand the power of plants. Since antiquity, medicinal herbs have been used to re-lieve throbbing headaches and heal minor cuts, scrapes, and burns. They can provide a surge of stamina or kick your digestive system into gear. Certain herbs assist your immune system in re-ducing fevers and fighting parasites. Some brighten your mood; others spice up your sex life. Still others help you with emotional stress.

Many prescription and over-the-counter products contain medicinal ingredients that are derived from, or similar to, those found in plants. For instance, acetylsalicylic acid, better known as aspirin, is similar to salicin, a pain reliever found in willow bark. Progesterone-like substances for birth control pills were derived from compounds found in Mexican yams.

Respect the medicinal powers of herbs. "Definitely treat herbs as you do medicine," says Mindy Green, a founding and professional member of the American Herbalists Guild, director of educational services for the Herb Research Foundation in Boulder, Colorado, and coauthor of *Aromatherapy: A Complete Guide to the Healing Art.*

Although most herbs are safe with few or no side effects, herbal experts caution that some can be toxic if taken in the wrong form or in large quantities. Especially when you're using an herb for the first time, it's wise to begin with the lowest recommended dosage. And watch for side effects before you consider increasing the amount, says Angela Stengler, N.D., a naturopathic physician and herbal author in Oceanside, California.

Comfrey, for example, is excellent when used externally as a poultice for sprains and bruises, but it can cause cancer or liver damage if ingested.

Choose the herb that's right for you. Before you buy an herb, make sure it's suitable for the condition you're treating.

"When someone wants to use herbs for the first time, I recommend that they try one herb for a specific need instead of buying a half-dozen," says Dr. Stengler. "See how your body interacts with this herb. Is it giving you the de-

WOMAN TO WOMAN
She Banishes Bad Feelings

What would you do if you were a woman alone, deep in a mountainous Central American jungle, and the relatives of the local medicine man started showing open envy and hostility toward you? That was the situation in which 57-year-old Rosita Arvigo, a doctor of naprapathy (a form of chiropractic), international herbal lecturer, and master herbalist, found herself. She had settled in Belize in 1981 to study herbal medicine. There she apprenticed herself to Don Eligio Panti, a traditional Mayan healer-priest, who taught her the ways of herbs. It was his relatives who came to resent her. And it was he who showed her what to do. This is her story.

Although I spend much of my time growing healing botanicals and operating the Ix Chel Tropical Research Farm in Belize, I do a fair amount of traveling worldwide to educate people about the benefits of herbs.

I learned much of what I know about those benefits during the 17 years I spent studying with my wonderful teacher, Don Eligio Panti, a Mayan shaman who lived to be 103 years old. He taught me many things, but one of his first lessons was how to ward off destructive emotions.

When I first began meeting with my teacher, his family did not take kindly to me. Here I was, a stranger from a foreign land, an interloper, trespassing into their world and getting all the attention from their relative. Their feelings toward me were intense and frightening. They were jealous, full of envy.

Envy is an emotion without merit. Whether you're on the receiving end or wishing you could be more like so-and-so, envy only spurs feelings of discouragement and resentment.

Soon I began having nightmares and feelings of depression.

sired effect? Are there any side effects? Get to know the herb. What it looks like. How it works."

Know the versatility of herbs. Certain herbs provide both culinary delight and medicinal benefits. Fresh cloves of garlic liven a dish of

I found myself wanting to give up and move away. But I didn't. Instead, I took a lesson from my teacher.

I had seen Don Eligio use the herb rue to deal with envy under other circumstances. Now it was time to put that lesson to a practical test. Twice every day, just before meals, I squeezed nine small branches of rue into a glass of water and drank it. Soon, my nightmares and depression went away, and I was able to cope until the relatives' envy lessened and they accepted me. I will always be grateful to Don Eligio for that lesson.

Now, I consider rue an herb of grace. It's my buddy. Whenever I travel from my home in the rain forest to the United States or some other place in the world to present herbal workshops, I never forget to tuck some in my pocket. Then, whenever I find myself feeling envious of someone— or becoming the object of their envy—I simply reach into my pocket and give the tiny branches a gentle squeeze to re- mind me to let go of the jealousy and not let it consume me.

Rue is easy to find. It commonly grows along roadsides and does well in pots, indoors during the winter. It's a shrubby herb, no taller than three feet, with a strong scent and yellow flower. Rue can irritate the gastrointestinal tract, and you shouldn't use it if you have kidney problems. It can also irritate your skin and increase your sensitivity to the sun. You can drink it to fight emotions like envy, discourage- ment, and feelings of upset, or you can soak the leaves in al- cohol and use it as a liniment to relieve muscle aches. Use it fresh, and don't boil it.

If ever you find yourself emotionally upset or facing a con- frontation, remember what traditional healers from Central America and the Caribbean have said for generations: "When you don't know what to do, get that rue."

Know the limitations of herbs. Herbs work effectively for the occa- sional headache or sleep-interrupted night, colds, the flu, or the rash you got from hiking in woods laced with poison ivy. Botanical medicine can even contribute to optimal health when it's used correctly as part of an overall wellness program, says Dr. Stengler. But botanicals alone cannot be expected to solve all health prob- lems, especially major ones, such as heart disease, high blood pressure, dia- betes, or cancer.

Don't expect miracles. Herbs, like vitamins and prescriptions, won't make up for lack of exercise or poor eating habits. Herbs work best when you incorporate nutritious foods and regular exercise into your lifestyle.

Learning the Herbal Lingo

It could be a shopper's nightmare: aisles and aisles of herbs. Some in tiny glass bottles. Others in capsules. Some fresh, some dried. Still others are in teas, chewing gum, throat lozenges, salves, and ear drops.

On the other hand, if you know where to begin, it could be a shopper's paradise.

Let's begin right here, by learning the benefits and drawbacks of selecting herbs in five basic forms: tinctures, teas, cap- sules, powders, and poultices.

Take a tincture. Tinctures are extracts made by steeping herbs in alcohol. They work best when you need quick absorption. "They are es- pecially helpful for women who have trouble ab-

clams and linguine, but garlic may also help pre- vent major cardiovascular disease when used in appropriate amounts over specified periods of time. Sage is another culinary spice that, when used medicinally, works effectively as a gargle for sore throats.

WOMEN ASK WHY

I love cooking with herbs and use them all the time, so why do I need to take herbal supplements to get the benefits of herbal healing?

It's a matter of arithmetic. Many herbs offer culinary delight when sipped in teas, sprinkled on foods, tossed in salads, or cooked in stews, but in most instances, the amounts are far too small to give you any real medicinal benefits.

Let's consider two popular herbs: garlic and ginkgo.

A crushed clove of garlic added to your favorite pasta sauce delivers an inviting aroma and a satisfying taste, but studies show that you must eat at least one and up to five cloves of garlic per day, each containing about 5,000 micrograms of allicin, to lower your blood pressure and cholesterol. Who's going to do that? It's unrealistic. You can gain the same therapeutic benefits much more easily and conveniently (and avoid bad breath) by swallowing standardized extract garlic capsules or tinctures.

If you're looking to improve your memory and circulation, ginkgo is an ideal herb choice. But, again, supplements provide more medicinal value than a cup of tea made with fresh or dried ginkgo.

Most studies indicate that you need to take 60 to 240 milligrams (24 percent standardized extract) to achieve the medicinal benefits needed to sharpen your memory and enhance circulation. To match that amount, you'd need to drink up to 15 cups of ginkgo tea a day. Who has the time, let alone the taste, to do this?

Eating herbs for flavor is fine. They provide a nutritional plus to diets. For treating specific health conditions, however, herbs eaten in foods cannot match the therapeutic values of supplements.

Expert consulted
Angela Stengler, N.D.
Naturopathic physician
Oceanside, California

sorbing nutrients because of digestive problems," explains Dr. Stengler. "Tasting the herb stimulates digestion and body processes."

Depending on the herb, you can use a tincture internally or externally. Most tinctures are made with diluted alcohol (100 proof) or a mixture of 50 percent ethanol and 50 percent water. Nonalcoholic tinctures made with glycerin are also available. Either type can be taken directly by mouth or added to water, juice, or herbal tea for better palatability. When stored in a cool, dark place, a tincture can last for several years without losing strength. But they don't always taste great and are not routinely standardized.

Sip some tea. A popular way to take medicinal herbs is by drinking a small amount of fresh or dried herb in a steaming cup of tea. Most herbal teas contain high concentrations of volatile oils, but they take time to make and may not be as potent as tinctures or capsules.

To get the same memory-sharpening benefits from ginkgo tea that you would from a 180-milligram capsule of extract, you'd have to drink 15 cups, says Dr. Stengler.

Still, herbal teas have one huge advantage: They usually taste great. For your favorite herbal blends, consider buying herbs in bulk that have been organically grown and are free of commercial fertilizers. These herbs should smell fresh, be free of mold, and nearly match the color of fresh herbs. Store them in airtight containers away from sunlight.

Swallow a capsule. Herbs in capsule form are often standardized and offer convenience. If a person has difficulty swallowing pills, the capsules can be opened and the contents stirred into food or liquids. It takes the body longer to absorb a capsule than a tincture, however. And if there is no expiration date on the label, it can be difficult to judge freshness.

Sprinkle on powder. You can easily add herbs in powder form to food or beverages to provide a direct effect on the throat and gastrointestinal system. For example, adding a teaspoon of slippery elm to your morning oatmeal will help soothe a sore throat or relieve heartburn, according to Dr. Stengler. The downside of powders is that they are hard to standardize unless the powder comes from a capsule.

Apply a poultice. A poultice is a layer of crushed herb, fresh or dried, that is dampened and applied directly to the affected area of the body. Normally, a layer of cotton, such as cheesecloth, is placed between the herb and the skin. A poultice provides relief to external parts of the body only. For instance, if you burned your forearm, a calendula poultice would speed the healing of your skin. You would not use a poultice, however, to relieve a cold, says Dr. Stengler.

Decoding the Label

Package labels are supposed to make our lives easier. The labels on

---

THE HERBAL KITCHEN
Infusions and Decoctions

Sipping any steamy, hot cup of herbal tea can make you feel cozy, warm, and wonderful, but if you want to maximize its medicinal strength, there are two ways of preparing it: You can make an infusion or a decoction.

You make an infusion by steeping one ounce of fresh or dried herb leaves and flowers in one pint of boiling water. Herbalists regard infusions as simple rituals that unite a healer (you) and a healing substance (the herb) with a healing intention ("I want to get a good night's sleep," for instance).

A decoction is similarly created by simmering one ounce of tough herb parts (usually the roots, bark, dried berries, or seeds) for each pint of boiling water, usually for about 10 to 20 minutes. This long simmering process coaxes out the plant's medicinal properties.

To make an infusion to combat a cold, for example, place one teaspoon of fresh or dried astragalus in a glass, ceramic, or plastic infuser; a cloth tea bag; or a metal tea ball. Place in a teapot. In a separate kettle or pot, boil one cup of water. Pour the boiling water over the herbs, then cover and steep for 10 to 15 minutes. The lid prevents the herb's essential oils from escaping in the steam. Drink daily for a few months before and during the cold and flu season.

To make a decoction to curb a cough, place one teaspoon of fresh or dried licorice root, crushed or chopped, in a glass or stainless steel pot with a lid. Add one cup of water. Bring to a full boil, then reduce the heat to the lowest setting, and let the root simmer gently for about 20 minutes. Keep the pot covered. Strain the decoction through a fine-mesh plastic strainer into a pint or quart glass jar. Press the herbs in the strainer with the back of a wooden spoon to extract more of its liquid. Licorice is an anti-inflammatory, antiviral herb that soothes coughs. You can drink up to three cups per day.

herbal products don't. By law, they cannot carry medicinal claims or post possible side effects unless these have been proven in tests that cost millions of dollars and require years to undertake.

Since plants can't be patented, it doesn't make financial sense for companies to spend millions of dollars establishing evidence that ginger, for instance, helps in digestive complaints. The Food and Drug Administration classifies herbal products that have not been through its drug premarket approval process as dietary supplements, not drugs.

Even with vague labeling, however, consumers can navigate effectively through the herbal product aisle with the following tips.

Learn both the botanical and common name of the herb. Knowing the botanical, or Latin, name gives you an extra edge when making a purchase. It guarantees you're buying the right type of herb for your needs. Depending on where you live, an herb answers to several names. The hormone-balancing herb that eases menstrual discomfort is known as chasteberry as well as vitex. And some herbs, such as echinacea, come in several types. The savvy shopper seeking relief from a cold would know to ask for *Echinacea purpurea* and not *Echinacea angustifolia*, according to Dr. Stengler, because the former has been the subject of more research.

Buy brands that are standardized. This assures that you will get the same dose of the active ingredient every time. It says so on the label. The potency of herbs can vary from batch to batch, plant to plant, place to place, and time to time. Buying standardized avoids guesswork.

REAL-LIFE SCENARIO
More Is Not Better

Kathy, age 49, has been stocking her medicine cabinet with healing herbs since she suffered a painful urinary tract infection five years ago. Now she takes about 12 herbs a day: angelica for digestive problems, ginkgo for more energy, kava kava as a mood booster, plantain and bearberry to prevent bladder and urinary tract infections, mullein and echinacea for yeast infections, evening primrose for breast tenderness, valerian for insomnia, sarsaparilla and Oregon grape to clear up her skin, and lemon balm to reduce tension. This is at no small cost. She spends nearly $80 a month on herbs! So she wasn't too pleased when she recently read that certain herbs lose their effectiveness when they're mixed together. Still, she feels better than ever! Could it be the herbs or is she just wasting her money?

When it comes to herbal remedies, less is often best. Kathy may feel great, but taking a dozen herbs a day is probably not the reason. She could get the same results with only a few herbs—and she'd improve the balance in her savings account at the same time.

What Kathy has read is true: Certain herbs can cancel each other out, but that's not the only bug in her herbal program. She may not be doing herself any favors by taking some herbs over an extended period. For example, certain immune-system boosters, such as echinacea, can lose their

---

But be aware that most herbs aren't available in standardized form, so you may need to rely upon other factors to help make your selection.

Look for expiration dates and safety seals. To ensure full potency of capsules, buy only products that post an expiration date. Without a date, you cannot be sure how old the capsules are. Also, buy products with safety seals for added protection.

Seek the recommended dosage. Manufacturer's recommended dosages vary from one product to another, so it's a good practice to check the label before taking the herb. Note if effectiveness when taken every day for too long a time. Other herbs, such as kava kava, can cause side effects when used for weeks on end. Even if none of this applies to the herbs she's taking, Kathy has no way of knowing which ones are actually making her feel better and which ones are not helping her at all.

A better strategy for Kathy would be to limit herself to just a few herbs that can treat more than one problem at a time. Mullein, for example, can help her yeast and urinary tract infections, her digestive complaints, and her skin problems.

Kathy should also consider that the best remedies for some health problems do not come from herb gardens. For instance, her tendency to get infections may be related to what she eats. She could be getting too much sugar in her diet, which could be suppressing her immune system. Or maybe she's not eating enough vitamin- or mineral-rich foods. As for her insomnia, tension, and lack of energy, Kathy could improve all three with exercise, yoga, or relaxation techniques such as meditation or deep breathing.

The bottom line: A combination of just a few herbs and other natural therapies can help Kathy feel great without spending a fortune.

Expert consulted
Amy Rothenberg, N.D.
Naturopathic physician
Enfield, Connecticut

the instructions tell you to take the herb with meals or in between meals.

Choose organic. The label should clearly state if the product was made free of chemical fertilizers. Most certified organic products are processed according to standards outlined in the California Organic Food Act of 1990. Some products include that information on their labels as well.

Check the ingredients. The label should display the amount of every active ingredient. Make sure that the product does not contain any ingredient you may be allergic to. Also, check for any fillers or preservatives that may have been added.

Choose single-herb products. You may like that multivitamin you take every day, but when it comes to selecting herbs, experts recommend that you avoid buying multi-herb products. By taking several herbs blended into one product, such as a capsule, you may get inadequate doses of each.

Buy proven herb brands. Select herbs from brands that have been tested. These brands are backed by solid research. Examples include Kwai garlic, Ginkgold ginkgo, Thisilyn milk thistle, and Kira St. John's wort.

Look for cautions. Many reputable manufacturers will list special precautions, such as the best time to take the product (with meals or in between) and when you should avoid it (if you're pregnant or have a specified medical condition, for example).

Steer clear of miracle claims. Avoid buying herbal products that claim they contain "secret formulas" or "miracle cures." If an herb sounds too good to be true—and lacks scientific backing—it probably is.

Find the manufacturer. By law, the manufacturer's address must be included on the label. Manufacturers who provide telephone numbers and Web site addresses build their credibility with consumers.

Using Herbs Safely and Wisely

If by now you've ventured out and purchased the teas, tinctures, and capsules you need, congratulations! You've taken the first step. Proper use of your herbs is the second. To ensure a safe and effective experience, herbal experts offer these tips.

10 EASY-TO-GROW WINDOWSILL HERBS

There's one sure way to guarantee that your herbs will be fresh: Grow your own. You don't have to own a tract of farmland or live in a tropical climate. In fact, you don't even have to go outdoors. There's nothing more warming on a dark, snowy winter's day than the sight of something alive, green, and growing in your kitchen or living room.

Luckily, many herbs love an indoor climate and a pot of their own. Following are 10 medicinal herbs that do well in pots or windowsills, according to Mindy Green, a founding and professional member of the American Herbalists Guild, director of educational services for the Herb Research Foundation in Boulder, Colorado, and coauthor of *Aromatherapy: A Complete Guide to the Healing Art*.

"All of these are easy to grow, especially thyme and rosemary, which are great culinary herbs," says Green. "Anytime you fertilize a plant you intend to use for eating, use organic fertilizer because it doesn't contain chemicals."

In addition, keep the following preparation tips in mind.

- Select pots that have drainage holes and are at least 12 inches in diameter.
- Choose herbal plants that are 3 to 4 inches in height.
- Use porous potting mix and organic fertilizer.

Herb	Growing Tip	Medicinal Use	Part Used (Form)
Calendula	Full sun	Minor burns, rashes	Flowers, leaves (ointment)
Chamomile	Full sun to part shade	Insomnia, indigestion	Leaves (tea)
Feverfew	Full sun to part shade	Migraines	Leaves (fresh leaf)
Lavender	Full sun	Stress	Flowers (tea)
Lemon balm	Full sun to part shade	Stress	Leaves (fresh leaf)
Lemon thyme	Full sun to part shade	Congestion from colds	Leaves (tea)
Nasturtium*	Full sun; keep moist	Colds	Flowers (tea) or fresh (salads)
Peppermint	Full sun to part shade; keep moist	Headaches, indigestion	Leaves (tea, salve)
Rosemary	Full sun	Indigestion, nasal congestion	Leaves (tea, salve)
St. John's wort	Full sun to part shade	Bruises	Oil (external)

*Use sparingly. Nasturtium can irritate your stomach.

Use herbs only when needed. Home herbal remedies should only be used when necessary and only in appropriate amounts. This is not an area where a "more is better" philosophy applies. For example, echinacea works most effectively when taken at the onset of a cold to lessen its severity. But taking echinacea every day all year long may lessen its potency.

Rely on knowledgeable experts. Learn about herbs and talk them over with either your doctor or some other qualified health care practitioner who has training and experience in using herbs medicinally. She can be an M.D. or D.O. (medical doctor or doctor of osteopathy) trained in herbal medicine or an N.D. (naturopathic physician) trained in botanical medicine. She can also be simply an herbalist who knows the historical and current uses of herbs, understands how herbs work in our bodies, and often prepares herbal products for her clients, as long as she is open to coordinating your care with your physician.

Several organizations can provide you with names of qualified herbal practitioners in your area. These organizations include the American Herbalists Guild, P. O. Box 70, Roosevelt, UT 84066; the American Association of Naturopathic Physicians, 601 Valley Street, Suite 105, Seattle, WA 98109-4229; the National Commission for Certification for Acupuncture and Oriental Medicine, 11 Canal Center Plaza, Suite 300, Alexandria, VA 22314; and the American Holistic Medical Association, 6728 Old McLean Village Drive, McLean, VA 22101.

Know when to stop. Pay close attention to instructions on how long to take an herb. Some suggest you take a break for several weeks or months before resuming. Others you can take safely every day. Sometimes the recommended time depends upon the condition. You should expect some improvement in an acute condition such as a cold or the flu within 24 to 48 hours, says Dr. Stengler.

If the condition is chronic, such as arthritis or menopausal hot flashes, you may need to observe your symptoms for up to two months to feel any difference, she says. If your health condition does not improve after using the herbal remedy for a reasonable amount of time, seek medical help. Certainly, see your doctor if your condition worsens.

Keep your doctor informed. According to the *Journal of the American Medical Association*, 15 million Americans take herbs and prescription medicine at the same time. But 60 percent fail to tell their doctors that they are taking herbal remedies. Inform your doctor so that she can be on the lookout for possible drug-herb interactions.

Store herbs properly. Place dried herbs in airtight glass containers and store them in a cool, dark place. They will retain their potency for up to six months this way. For tinctures, using dark glass bottles will guarantee potency for several years. As for capsules, check for an expiration date and store them in a closed jar away from heat and sunlight.

Feel-Good Therapies

The fundamental uses of herbs are three: healing, cooking, and having fun.

That's right. *Having fun.* It's not all serious business. Herbs can heal you, but they can also bring you lots of enjoyment. Think about how they stir the senses—smell, touch, taste, sight. Imagine the lingering aroma of a lavender essential oil candle; the silky, rich sensation of a rose-infused massage oil; the sugary sweet taste of angelica candy; the bright, beautiful colors of a floral potpourri.

Still, they're actually medicines, aren't they? Well, that depends on your point of view. Herbs have a healing effect, but when was the last time a bottle of aspirin brought the words "pampering" and "self-indulgence" to mind?

It's true that, for some people, modern herbalism has simply become a substitute for traditional medicine. Think of all they're missing. They treat their bodies, but what about their minds and their spirits? Herbs can enrich people's daily lives in so many more ways, says herbalist Rosemary Gladstar, director of the Sage Mountain Herbal Education Center in

East Barre, Vermont, and author of *Herbal Healing for Women.*

Open yourself to a new world and experiment with all the different facets of herbology. Treat yourself to an herbal foot massage, cook up some herbal candies, cool down with a relaxing herbal-scented spritzer. In other words, have fun!

Aromatherapy

Through the senses of touch and smell, aromatherapy may help to erase the physical, emotional, and spiritual roadblocks women face every day. It uses essential oils, which are extremely concentrated aromatic oils distilled from plants. "It literally takes hundreds of pounds of plant material to produce a small amount of essential oil," Gladstar says.

People who practice aromatherapy say that each essential oil has specific healing properties. For instance, the scent of peppermint oil alleviates indigestion and nausea, rosemary treats lung congestion and sore throats, and sandalwood counters inflammation and hemorrhoids.

WAITING TO INHALE

In the art of aromatherapy, choosing which essential oils to use is only the first part of your preparation. You also have to decide how you want to disperse the aroma into the air or onto your body. Choose the method that is most appealing to you.

Aromatherapy companies have devised a wide range of devices to help you—from the efficient to the decorative. "There's something for everyone and for every price range," says herbalist Rosemary Gladstar, director of the Sage Mountain Herbal Education Center in East Barre, Vermont, and author of *Herbal Healing for Women*.

Here's a quick description of some popular and easy-to-use aromatherapy products.

Diffusers. Diffusers heat essential oils and spread their scent into the air. A basic ceramic diffuser (A) has a saucer at the top into which you drop oil and water. Directly underneath the saucer is a votive candle. The candle warms the oil and water, emitting essential oil vapors into the room. A more complex electronic diffuser (B) uses an air pump and an atomizer. For aromatherapy in your car, you can buy a diffuser that plugs into your cigarette lighter (C). The lighter socket heats up the oil, creating a relaxing refuge during a traffic jam or a rough commute.

Lamp rings. A lamp ring diffuser is a small ring made of ceramic that fits around the lightbulb of a lamp. You place the essential oils and water inside the ring. Heat generated by the bulb warms and diffuses the oils.

Mists. Mists are essential oil mixtures in spray bottles. You can buy them or make them yourself by mixing the oils, vodka, and distilled water. They can be sprayed in the air to scent a room or sprayed on your body.

Candles. Aromatherapy candles come in many different sizes and types. You can buy a candle scented with just one specific oil or purchase a candle made with a mixture specially created to promote a specific mood, such as relaxation, sensuality, or meditation.

Avoid rosemary if you have hypertension or epilepsy.

According to aromatherapists, this aromatic art works in two ways. First, it operates through inhalation. We've all experienced scents that influence our moods and emotions. Aromatherapy goes one step further. The theory is that specific scents trigger more than just feelings; they also incite internal chemical reactions that can enhance your immune system or reduce tension, says Mindy Green, a founding and professional member of the American Herbalists Guild (AHG), director of educational services for the Herb Research Foundation in Boulder, Colorado, and coauthor of *Aromatherapy: A Complete Guide to the Healing Art.*

Second, essential oils work topically, entering your body through your skin. To use oils in this way, pour them into baths, add them to massage oils, or apply them with compresses. "It isn't just the odor. There can be 500 different compounds in one oil. It has therapeutic properties that affect our entire systems," Gladstar says.

Many women turn to aromatherapy because of its simplicity. To get started, purchase 100 percent natural essential oils. Start your collection, Gladstar says, with three basic oils that have wide ranges of application: peppermint, chamomile, and lavender. Peppermint treats stomach problems, headaches, congestion, and muscle spasms, and it can be used as a natural stimulant. Chamomile may reduce indigestion, premenstrual syndrome, muscle inflammation, stress, and insomnia. Lavender is a wonderful emotional healer; it helps treat nervousness, exhaustion, insomnia, irritability, and even depression.

People with sensitive skin can have allergic reactions to essential oils, even when they're used externally. To be sure you're not one of them, first do a patch test. Put 10 to 12 drops of essential oil in an ounce of massage oil or unscented body lotion. Dab a bit of this mix on an inconspicuous place, such as your inner arm or on the back of your neck at the hairline. Over the next 12 hours, check for redness or itching. If either occur, use a weaker solution or try another oil.

Because they're so concentrated, essential oils can be toxic if you ingest them, so don't take them internally. It's also easy to overdo them with even a small amount, so always dilute any oil before applying it to the skin. Dilute essential oils with carrier oils, which are neutral, nonaromatic oils such as almond, jojoba, or grapeseed oils.

Here are some suggested recipes for using essential oils: For massage/body oils, 10 to 12 drops (from a standard medicine dropper) per ounce of carrier oil; for baths, 3 to 15 drops per bathtub; for inhalants, 3 to 5 drops per bowl of hot water; for room sprays, 20 drops per four ounces of water; for compresses, 5 drops per cup of water.

Baths/Hydrotherapy

People have been tapping into the healing powers of water for at least 6,000 years. Cold baths energize and stimulate. Room-temperature bathwater has been called nature's finest tranquilizer. The classic hot bath eases muscle spasms and relaxes the body and mind. Even ice and steam can bring comfort to a variety of everyday ailments.

Nothing can make you feel better than a long, hot bath can—nothing but a long, hot bath accentuated with herbs and essential oils, that is. "Baths are one of my favorite things. Therapeutically, it is like immersing your body in a giant cup of tea," Gladstar says. From the water, your skin absorbs the healing and soothing properties of herbs. They enhance the water's ability to relax you, soothe sore muscles, rejuvenate dried skin, and ease congestion from a cold.

To make an herbal bath, start with a strong tea. Place two or three handfuls of an herb or herbal mixture into two to three quarts of boiling water. Cover it tightly; let it cool to room temperature, and then strain it. Pour the herbal tea into a full tub of water, says Green.

Which herbs are good for baths? Just about any one, as long as it has a pleasant aroma, Green says. Avoid using large amounts of "hot" herbs like clove, cinnamon, ginger, or cayenne, she cautions. They can irritate the skin. For a beginner, she recommends experimenting with calming and sweet-smelling herbs, such as lemon balm, chamomile, rose, or lavender.

To use essential oils in a bath, Green suggests starting with geranium, orange, or lavender. You can use 3 drops of orange and up to 10 drops for geranium and lavender. For an ailment such as a cold, use 5 to 8 drops of eucalyptus oil. To get the full effect of an herbal bath, Green suggests soaking for at least 20 minutes.

Orange oil is phototoxic—if you use it, even diluted, in areas of skin that are exposed to the sun, it can cause uneven pigmentation. So reserve it for times when you won't be going out immediately into the sun. Don't use eucalyptus oil for more than two weeks. It's best added to one teaspoon of vegetable oil, then added to the bath.

WOMEN ASK WHY

Why is it that I can lose five pounds in a few minutes by having an herbal wrap, but I can't lose that much in a whole week of dieting?

An herbal wrap acts like a sponge on a wet surface: It sucks the moisture right out of your body. That's why some herbalists recommend it to draw out toxins such as caffeine and nicotine.

During a wrap, you'll lie still while you're swaddled in herb-soaked towels. Some therapists will also cover you with plastic. You'll start to feel warm and cozy. The tight wrap and the warmth will make you sweat profusely, which is how it draws water out of you.

Losing five pounds of water isn't difficult. Your body is made of 65 percent fluids, so it has plenty to spare. Unfortunately, it won't stay lost for long. Those five pounds will probably show up on your scale again within 24 hours of treatment.

Some people claim that a wrap will help you lose inches and shrink fat cells, but that's nonsense. Just as you have probably heard over and over again, losing weight is a matter of diet and exercise. It may take longer than an herbal wrap, but it's the only way to make sure those pounds are gone for good.

Expert consulted
Jenny McFeely
Member of Britain's National Institute
of Medical Herbalists
Professional member of the American
Herbalists Guild
Scottsdale, Arizona

If you don't have time to languish in a bath, you can still enjoy the soothing effects of herbs and water by making an herbal salt scrub to use in the shower, Gladstar says. Buy some natural sea salt at a health food store and pour it into a

THE HERBAL KITCHEN
Cooling Herbal-Scented Waters

How would you like to have your own portable oasis right in your pocketbook? There's nothing like spraying your body with some cool, herbal-scented water to take the edge off a tough, exhausting day or hot, muggy weather.

Sprays made with peppermint, lemon balm, and cucumber oil work especially well since they are naturally cool and refreshing, says herbalist Rosemary Gladstar, director of the Sage Mountain Herbal Education Center in East Barre, Vermont, and author of *Herbal Healing for Women*. With a few simple ingredients and a little bit of time, you can make your own. Keep some in your purse, some in your car, and some in your office. That way, you'll always have it on hand.

Purchase a four-ounce dark bottle with a twist-off spray pump at a beauty supply store. Using a small funnel, pour one tablespoon of vodka into the bottle. The alcohol acts as a preservative and keeps the cooling water from going bad. Using the funnel, pour distilled water into the bottle until it almost reaches the top. With a dropper, add three to five drops of essential oils. To enhance the cooling effect, use peppermint, lemon balm, orange, or cucumber essential oils. Shake it before each use. It should keep indefinitely. Don't use it on broken skin or spray it in your eyes.

Peppermint oil and lemon balm may cause skin irritation or an allergic reaction in people with very sensitive skin.

your circulation. Your skin is glowing and soft. It is marvelous," Gladstar says.

Cough Medicines

Although it takes a bit of cooking time, there's something to be said for making your own cough medicine. Herbal cough syrups are herbal decoctions and infusions—basically teas made by a long, slow simmering process. They not only soothe harsh coughs but also give you that special sense of satisfaction that always seems to come when you create something from scratch. "You always make better medicine at home. You have much more control over quality, how strong it is, the flavors. You have your own good intentions in that medicine," Gladstar says.

Take one teaspoon every hour or so, says herbalist Betzy Bancroft, a member of the AHG and manager at Herbalist and Alchemist in Washington, New Jersey. You can make syrups from fennel, coltsfoot, licorice, mullein, marshmallow, or wild cherry bark.

To make the syrup, combine any of these herbs, in tincture form, in equal parts (except only one-half part wild cherry bark) plus an amount of honey to equal the combined tinctures. If you want more flavor, add one-half part fruit concentrate, which you can buy at a health food store. Store the mixture out of the refrigerator. Shake it well before using it.

Gladstar offers this recipe: First, you make an herb tea. For a cough medicine that will calm a hard, dry cough, mix one-half part valerian, one

wide-mouth glass jar. Leave about two inches of space at the top. Pour almond oil over the sea salt until the jar is nearly full, then add two to five drops of essential oil, preferably lavender or lemon balm. When you're taking your shower, grab a handful of the salt and vigorously rub your body with it. Be gentle if you have sensitive skin. Then proceed with your regular shower. "This is done in expensive spas. You wash off all the dead cells in your skin, and you stimulate part mullein, one part licorice root, and one part wild cherry bark. Crush or chop the herbs. Place four ounces of the mixture per quart of water in a glass or stainless steel pot. Bring the liquid to a full, rolling boil, and then reduce the heat to the lowest setting and let the decoction simmer for 10 to 20 minutes. Keep the pot covered so that the herb's essential oils don't escape. Steep overnight in the refrigerator.

To make the syrup, simmer the decoction down to a pint. This will give you a concentrated, thick tea. Strain out the herbs. Pour the liquid back into the pot. For each pint, add one cup of honey. Warm the honey and liquid together until they mix well. If you desire, add three to four tablespoons of brandy per half-pint. Brandy acts as a preservative and relaxes throat muscles. Refrigerated, the syrup should last a few weeks.

Flower Essences

It sounds like a commercial, but it's true: If you want to express your feelings to someone, whether of love, grief, regret, or joy, there's almost no better way to do it than with flowers. The connection between flowers and emotions seems eternal, and people who use flower essences take this idea deeper. They believe that certain flowers possess a special ability to heal emotional hurts. Whereas essential oils capture the physical healing power of plants, flower essences capture their emotional healing power. Consider

NATURAL SCENTS THAT ATTRACT THE OPPOSITE SEX

In an ancient Tantric ritual once practiced in India, a woman would be anointed with essential oils so that adoring men would worship her as a goddess.

Now it's your turn to be adored, don't you think?

Essential oils historically thought to mesmerize the opposite sex include:

- ❥ Rose. This flower's scent has been the inspiration for poets and lovers for centuries.
- ❥ Jasmine. In India, women scent their hair with jasmine, which is also known as moonlight of the grove.
- ❥ Ylang-ylang. Ylang-ylang means "flowers of flowers" and is thought to sharpen the senses.

"Of course, a scent that entices one person may be a turnoff to another. Ylang-ylang is considered an aphrodisiac, but it is much too heady and sweet for me," says Gail Ulrich, an herbalist, director of the Blazing Star Herbal School in Shelburne Falls, Massachusetts, and author of *Herbs to Boost Immunity*. "I prefer citrus and woodsy scents."

Which scents make your heart beat a little faster are really a matter of personal preference.

To get you started in the realm of odor and *amor*, try these enticing herbal recipes created by Mindy Green, a founding and professional member of the American Herbalists Guild, director of educational services for the Herb Research Foundation in Boulder, Colorado, and coauthor of *Aromatherapy: A Complete Guide to the Healing Art*. Add the essential oil drops to two ounces of water in a glass mist bottle. Shake well and spray them around your bedroom.

Wild about You
Three drops of jasmine
Nine drops of grapefruit
One drop of carrot seed

Don't Be Shy
Three drops of rose
Four drops of sandalwood
Six drops of mandarin

flower essences the "soul" of plants, Gladstar says.

To make a flower essence, place a perfect flower in a glass or crystal bowl filled with spring water. Then set the bowl on the ground near the mother plant. After a few hours in the sun, remove the flower with a small twig and add the water to a small bottle filled halfway with brandy.

The first flower essences created were the Bach Flower Remedies, discovered by British immunologist, bacteriologist, and pathologist Edward Bach, M.D. Dr. Bach believed that emotional distress is the underlying cause of physical illness. He also believed that flowers have the ability to treat emotional problems and, therefore, prevent or cure diseases.

Each of his 38 Bach flower essences is supposed to treat a specific emotional condition. For instance, the flower essence cerato helps people who have trouble making decisions and who constantly seek advice from others. Gentian aids those who get discouraged easily or who become filled with self-doubt after every small setback. Water violet is for people who like to be alone and who are independent, talented, capable, clever, calm, and self-reliant. It's interesting that many of the flowers Dr. Bach used are actually blossoming herbs.

You'll find flower essences in health food stores. Just trickle a few drops on your tongue or add a few drops to a small glass and slowly sip. You can also add some flower essence into your bathwater or pour a few drops into a spritzer bottle filled with water and keep it in your purse. Gladstar always takes a spray bottle of Rescue

Remedy—Dr. Bach's famous five-flower combination for relieving stress—with her when she flies. "I do it to keep centered and focused and happy," she says.

Candies and Lozenges

If flowers don't catch your interest, then how about candy? Herbal candies can be good for you, and they taste good, too. Some contain blends such as peppermint, thyme, sage elder,

---

REAL-LIFE SCENARIO
Can She Pamper Away Her Pain?

Marty, a 45-year-old office manager, always has a pounding tension headache by lunchtime, and her typing-intensive job causes muscle spasms in her back. Some days the pain is so bad that she practically hobbles to her car at quitting time. On top of that, she misses a few days of work every spring and fall to recover from a bad case of hay fever, which makes her constantly sneeze. Her doctor prescribed antihistamines, muscle relaxants, tranquilizers, and chiropractic adjustments. But she's still sneezing and in pain. She's now seeing an herbalist who recommends massage with essential oils. Marty's willing to give it a try, but she's a little skeptical. Could this one treatment be the answer to all her health problems?

It may sound too good to be true, but Marty may have just made a wonderful discovery. A little bit of pressure applied to the right places on her face and scalp can melt away the pain of a tension headache in minutes. And while this hands-on therapy won't eliminate Marty's seasonal allergies altogether, it can ease her hay fever symptoms in several ways.

For one thing, massage helps strengthen the immune system by reducing stress—and a strong immune system is less likely to overreact to allergens, such as molds or pollen. In addition, massage also helps relieve sinus pressure and unclog a stuffy head by loosening phlegm.

Massage can be even more effective when it's done with essential oils. Tiger balm, peppermint oil, and tea tree oil, for example, may reduce swelling in your sinuses and help open nasal passages. But Marty needs to be cautious: Some people are allergic to essential oils and could develop a rash when they're applied to the skin. To be on the safe side, she should make sure her massage therapist does what's called a patch test to see whether the oils will irritate her skin. During the test, the therapist will place very small amounts of various substances on her skin to see if any redness or swelling appears.

As for Marty's back spasms, massage can untie these painful knots by relaxing the contracted muscles and increasing blood flow. For even better results, Marty could try using lavender in her massage. This essential oil has relaxing properties that can also help to soothe muscle spasms.

Soon Marty may realize that massage has other benefits as well. She may find that she's becoming more flexible, that she has healthier skin, and that her digestion has improved. Best of all, she'll start to feel pampered.

Expert consulted
Amber Ackerson, N.D.
Naturopathic physician and licensed massage
*   therapist*
Director of quality assurance for the nutrition
*   supply company Tyler Encapsulations*
Gresham, Oregon

and horehound, while others combine lemon with mint, essential oils, and even vitamin C. The old standby sore throat/cough drop contains the herb eucalyptus. Gladstar remembers when, as a child, she enjoyed Jump for Joy balls and horehound candies and lozenges made from powdered herbs.

You can find many of these candies at your local drugstore or health food store, but you can also make your own. Here's how: For candy, choose some herbs that have a pleasant taste or scent, perhaps angelica and fennel. Lozenges are just medicated candy. One combination that is effective against sore throats uses sage, fenugreek, licorice, or slippery elm, Bancroft says.

To make candy or lozenges, place one cup of a decoction or infusion designed for the illness you want to treat in a glass, ceramic, or stainless steel pan and add one-half cup honey or sugar. Simmer over low heat, stirring occasionally with a spatula or wooden spoon. Continue cooking the syrup until it is thick enough to coat the back of the spoon. Test it by dropping a small amount onto wax paper. As it cools, it should harden and hold its form.

Use one-half to one teaspoon of syrup for each candy or lozenge. After the candy has cooled and hardened, wrap each piece in plastic wrap, then store it all in a cool place. They will keep for several months.

Massage Oils

It is instinctive for us to touch ourselves or another person when we're in physical or emotional need. Without thinking, you rub your temples if you have a headache, knead your calves if they're cramped, and put your arm around someone's shoulder if she's troubled. That's why therapeutic massage works so well. It's an expression of a basic human impulse. "Massage itself is therapeutic. Everyone needs more touching—foot massage, hand massage, a back rub," Gladstar says.

By adding herbs to massage oils, you can intensify this nondrug approach to relieving tension, reducing stress, and easing muscle pain. Certain herbs also help with skin care.

To make your massage oil, first choose a carrier oil. Good carrier oils for massage include almond, apricot, or grapeseed. Then decide which essential oil you want to use. For a relaxing massage, Gladstar recommends rose, lavender, chamomile, or comfrey. You can use them singly or mixed together.

For muscle pain and strains, Green suggests rosemary, juniper, and wintergreen. To loosen tight, cramped muscles, try sage. For dry skin, make a calendula massage oil.

After choosing your herb or herbs, place two ounces of dried herbs in a wide-mouth jar. Pour a pint of carrier oil over the mixture so that at least two inches of oil sits above the herbs, Gladstar says. Let it sit in a warm place and shake it every day for two weeks. Using a kitchen strainer or a cheesecloth, strain the oil. Store it in your refrigerator and warm it in a pan on the stove before using it.

The oil should last for several months, but not more than a year. If you like, you can also add a few drops of an essential oil to the mixture. Use about 10 to 12 drops of essential oil to each pint of carrier oil.

If you need the oil quickly, place the herbs and oil in a double boiler, Gladstar says. Cover it with a tight-fitting lid and bring it to a slow simmer. Slowly heat the mixture for 45 minutes. Check frequently to make sure the oil doesn't get too hot. If it starts bubbling or smoking, reduce the heat. Strain the oil and then add a drop or two of an essential oil to enhance the aroma.

Skin Care/Topical Beauty

Beautiful skin. Every woman wants it. In 1400 B.C., an Egyptian queen was buried with tiny pots that are believed to have held her precious cosmetic creams and oils. During the second century, the ancient Roman doctor Galen created a recipe for face cream, possibly the first ever recorded. Made up of oils, wax, and water, it is a formula some herbalists still use today.

For many women, it makes perfect sense to use natural products to promote their own natural beauty. "Your skin is your largest organ of elimination and assimilation. Using herbs nourishes the skin and helps develop a radiance," Gladstar says.

Natural ingredients are useful in almost every aspect of your beauty regimen. Cleansing soaps, facial steams, shampoos, astringents, creams, and beauty masks all originate from herbs and plants. Many commercial skin care and cosmetic products contain herbs, but that doesn't make them true herbal formulas.

"A lot of herbs are being used in products that are not natural by any means. You need to be discriminating," Gladstar says. Look for products that contain natural ingredients that you recognize. Too many chemical names in the ingredient list is a tip-off that the product is not natural.

If you have skin that has lost its luster, herbalists recommend two time-honored techniques: cleansing scrubs and toners.

Some herbal scrubs are gentle enough to use every day on your face and body. They clean, soften, exfoliate, remove dirt-filled oils, and smell great.

Herbalists say that it's important to apply a toner after scrubbing. Versatile and fragrant, toners promote circulation, soften, and help restore the skin's natural acid mantle. This slightly acidic surface, which is often washed away by harsh soaps, plays a crucial part in protecting your skin from bacterial invasions.

To restore vibrancy to your skin, incorporate this two-step herbal strategy into your daily beauty regimen with an easy-to-make scrub and toner.

You'll need the following equipment: a food processor, clean coffee grinder, or blender; a large mixing bowl; a wire whisk; and a quart jar with a tight-fitting lid. You'll also need the following ingredients: one cup of ground oatmeal from rolled oats, one-quarter cup of ground almonds or poppy seeds, two cups of cosmetic clay, and one-eighth cup of ground dried lavender, roses, calendula, comfrey, or chamomile (or any combination of these herbs).

To make your scrub, first grind the oatmeal to a fine powder in the food processor, coffee grinder, or blender. Place the powder in the mixing bowl. Then grind the almonds or poppy seeds to a fine powder and add to the bowl. Next, add the clay and herbs to the combined ground oatmeal and seeds. Mix thoroughly with the wire whisk. Pour the mixture into the jar and put on the lid. (The mixture can be stored for a year.)

To use your scrub, pour out two tablespoons of the mixture into your hands, add water to make a thin paste, and scrub your face and upper body gently. The selected ingredients soothe your skin, lift away dirt, exfoliate, and even clean your pores. Rinse and follow with a toner.

To make your toner, you'll need the following equipment: a pint-size glass jar with a tight-fitting lid, a fine-mesh strainer, a large mixing bowl, a measuring cup, a funnel, and eight plastic bottles with tight-fitting lids. You'll also need two cups of apple-cider vinegar, witch hazel, distilled water, and your choice of one or several herbs from the following list: comfrey leaves, plantain, calendula, red roses, chamomile, nettles, lemon balm, lavender, scented geranium leaves, mullein, yarrow, rosemary, and thyme.

Start by packing your chosen herbs into the jar. (If you're using dried herbs, fill the jar halfway; if you're using fresh herbs, loosely layer them to the top of the jar.) Next, pour in the vinegar and close the lid tightly. Let the liquid steep for three to six weeks, then pour it through a strainer into a bowl. Add two tablespoons of witch hazel to the strained vinegar. Pour one-quarter cup of this mixture into each plastic bottle, and top each bottle with two cups of distilled water. Shake well before using.

The mixture will last for a year. Remember to refrigerate the bottles you aren't currently using. Don't worry if a slimy coating appears on the surface. Just remove it—it doesn't affect the quality of the toner. Apply the toner with a cotton ball or pad. You can also store it in a misting bottle and spritz your face and body whenever you need a pick-me-up.

Preparing an herbal facial steam is one of the easiest ways to treat your skin, and it does wonders. Bring two to three quarts of water to a boil in a large pot. Toss in a healthy handful of an herb or herbal mixture.

For dry to normal skin, Gladstar recommends chamomile, roses, comfrey, lavender, and calendula. For normal to oily skin, she suggests sage, comfrey, calendula, and rosemary. Cover the pot, and let the water simmer for a few minutes. After you remove the pot from the heat source, place it on a stable surface, cover your head with a large towel, and put your face about 12 inches over the steaming brew. Steam for five to eight minutes. When you're done, rinse your face with cold water and follow with a good moisturizing cream. Try this facial steam once a week, being careful not to spill the hot water.

Hair Rejuvenators

Want in on a little secret? Centuries before you could buy hair coloring in a box, women were washing away gray—naturally.

Natural dyes work like commercial shampoo-in color treatments, but they get their hue-changing power from compounds in plants, not from chemical coloring agents. As with all hair coloring, it's important to select an herbal gray-hider carefully, based on your original hair color and how much gray you want to cover.

For dark hair that's just beginning to sprout streaks of silver, a rinse with a strong cup of sage or rosemary tea can restore your original, deep shade, says Shatoiya de la Tour, an herbalist and founder of Dry Creek Herb Farm and Learning Center in Auburn, California. To make the tea, put two teaspoons of either herb in a cup of just-boiled water. Steep until cool, strain out the herbs, and use the liquid as a rinse after shampooing. Don't rinse this colored rinse out. Your hair should darken after several applications.

For hair that's brown, auburn, or medium to dark gray (not all-white), try this strong herbal tea rinse. To eight cups of boiling water add one-quarter cup each of dried nettles, sage, and rosemary; one-half cup of black walnut hulls; and two black tea bags, suggests beauty expert Stephanie Tourles, a licensed aesthetician in Hyannis, Massachusetts, and author of *The Herbal Body Book*. Steep for three hours and

---

MAKING A HENNA PASTE

You don't want to go gray, but you've heard the horror stories about red dye number this or yellow dye number that. Then henna might be just the thing for you. Fortunately, you don't have to travel halfway around the world to find it. Henna powders of all shades are readily available at health food stores and through mail-order catalogs.

Let herbalist Rosemary Gladstar, director of the Sage Mountain Herbal Education Center in East Barre, Vermont, and author of *Herbal Healing for Women*, guide you step-by-step in using henna paste for a new hue.

Here are some facts about henna.

- No matter what color you choose, all hennas will contain some red. So if you're blonde, expect red highlights.
- Unless your hair is super dirty, it's best to not shampoo your hair before applying the henna.
- After application, henna will seem to be a full shade brighter than you expect. But it will fade dramatically after the first washing.
- Henna shades last about two to three months.

Now, here's how to apply henna.

- Select the right amount of henna for your hair length—two to three ounces for short hair and four to six ounces for shoulder-length or longer hair.
- Mix the henna with boiling water to make a thick paste. Aim for a consistency similar to cooked oatmeal, not

---

strain. Then add two teaspoons of sweet almond or olive oil and chill the mix in the refrigerator. Wash and rinse your hair, then put on rubber gloves and apply one-half cup of this mixture. Let it sit for a minute. Don't rinse; just towel-dry your hair with a dark towel that won't show stains. Use this treatment daily for two weeks, then as desired, recommends Tourles.

You can enhance your natural hair color by artfully applying henna, an herbal hair coloring made from powdered privet leaves (for blonde too dry and not too runny. Let the paste cool before applying.

❧ Dampen hair thoroughly and towel-dry.

❧ Before applying henna, put on plastic gloves to avoid stains on your hands.

❧ Massage a small amount of olive or jojoba oil into your hair.

❧ Cover your hair completely with the henna paste. Your hair should feel like a thick helmet on your head.

❧ Cover your hair with a shower cap, plastic wrap, or plastic bag. Then hold it in place with a turban-wrapped towel.

❧ Depending on your shade of hair, leave the henna in for 30 minutes to two hours. The darker your hair shade, the longer you leave the henna on.

❧ Wash your hair with your normal shampoo and de-tangling rinse.

❧ Pick an old towel or T-shirt to dry your hair because the henna will leave stains.

❧ Let your hair air-dry before you brush.

❧ Remember, you won't see any shade differences until your hair is completely dry.

Note: If you have light-colored hair (blonde, light brown, silver), always choose a lighter shade of henna, such as neutral to strawberry blonde. Leave the henna in your hair for approximately 30 minutes. You might want to test it on a few strands before applying it to your entire head.

and red hair) or from powdered indigo (for black hair). Henna hair-coloring kits come in a wide variety of subtle shades. Choose a hue that accentuates your natural hair color.

Potpourri

In some circles, potpourri is referred to as recreational aromatherapy. Potpourri is a simple art, used more to make a room smell nice than to treat medical conditions. "Having a pleasant fragrance around you is really uplifting, especially since we are bombarded with so many nasty smells," Bancroft says.

Potpourri has become increasingly popular, with sprays and flower mixtures available at department stores. But some contain artificial ingredients and synthetic oils, which can be harsh on your skin and your senses. Since potpourri is easy to make, you may as well use the natural and safe scents Mother Nature gave us, Green says.

The simplest way to create potpourri is to make a sachet. Pick flowers from your garden or herbs that you like, dry and crush them, and place them in a small cloth bag. If you don't have a bag, sew two pieces of cloth together and stuff it with dried herbal mixtures, Bancroft says. Another easy potpourri technique is to simmer various herbs and plants in a pot of water on the stove. The scent will fill the air in moments. Popular plants used in potpourri include angelica, bay leaves, lemon balm, lavender, marjoram, and rosemary, although you can use whatever scents and herbs you enjoy.

PART TWO

Herbal
Know-How

50 Herbs Every Woman Should Know

How would you like to make friends with a plant? Or better yet, with 50 of them? Herbs won't feed your cat while you're off cruising the Caribbean, of course, but they will always be there for you when you need them most. They can protect, strengthen, relax, or invigorate you. They can spice up your meals, and they can lace the air around you with delicate scents. They're great to know.

So welcome to their domain. Make yourself at home. And don't be surprised if you find yourself feeling a natural connection with them. Women always have, for a very good reason: "Plants offer more affinity and, in general, work more gently on our female systems than pills and medications," says Jennifer Reid, N.D., a naturopathic physician in Gresham, Oregon.

Making new friends and developing relationships takes time, of course. And that's half the pleasure. When you first meet a new botanical, study it. Use it. Familiarize yourself with its shape, aroma, and healing powers. Feel how it interacts with your body before trying another, encourages Angela Stengler, N.D., a naturopathic physician and herbal author in Oceanside, California.

Each of the herbs you're about to meet has an enduring safety record, demonstrated effectiveness (often backed by scientific studies), preventive qualities, and popularity among the top herbal practitioners.

These 50 herbs can help in all the areas of your life. Some of them help rev up your body's immune engine against invading viruses. Others assist in cleansing key organs, such as the liver. Some help restore hormonal balance. For your needs as a woman, cramp bark can ease menstrual cramps, while black cohosh can cool menopausal hot flashes. For your emotional needs, St. John's wort can chase away mild depression. Peppermint can aid in digestion by reducing flatulence and abdominal cramps. For your beauty and pampering needs, it's hard to resist a relaxing lavender bath or a skin-cleansing herbal facial.

"Herbs nourish our entire being, not just the physical body. They nourish our cells with their nutrients, and they nourish our inner being with their strength and beauty," says herbalist Rosemary Gladstar, director of the Sage Mountain Herbal Education Center in East Barre, Vermont, and author of *Herbal Healing for Women.* "I encourage all women to build a strong relationship with herbs."

One note of caution: Many herbs, even those considered generally safe, can cause unwanted side effects in pregnant women, so if you're pregnant or suspect that you might be, it's a good idea to avoid using herbs regularly or in medicinal doses unless your obstetrician tells you otherwise. Experts also advise caution while breastfeeding, to ensure a safe supply of breast milk for your new baby.

Aloe

Aloe barbadensis
Also known as aloes; aloe vera

Regarded as a skin-soother since the days of ancient Egypt, this spiky, spiny plant appears in a wide variety of first-aid and hair-care products and cosmetics.

Highly regarded as nature's first line of treatment for skin irritations, minor cuts, and minor burns, aloe's transparent gel effectively hastens wound healing and promotes cell growth and attachment. Aloe shows potential healing qualities for psoriasis and frostbite.

For best results, herbalists recommend snapping off a lower aloe leaf near the center stalk, removing any spines, and then splitting the leaf in half. Scrape the oozing gel directly onto your wound. Fresh gel delivers greater healing power than first-aid products containing aloe.

WOMEN ASK WHY

If healing herbs have been around for thousands of years, why haven't I heard about them until recently?

Healing herbs slipped from their place in public awareness with the advent of modern medicines in the nineteenth century. Medicinal herbs are far from new, however. Take aloe, for example. Its medical uses date back some 4,000 years. The ancient Egyptians added aloe to the incense they used for embalming, and many scholars believe it was among the ointments used to embalm Christ.

Juice from the aloe plant was commonly taken as a laxative by the Greeks and Romans, and aloe gel was used in the first century to treat all kinds of ailments, including wounds, bruises, and skin irritations. In colonial times, a pharmacy in Virginia stocked aloe among its other medical supplies.

About 65 years ago, researchers discovered that aloe quickly and completely healed burns from x-rays and ultraviolet and gamma rays. Studies show that aloe gel speeds wound healing in several ways, but researchers have yet to identify the herb's active ingredient.

More recently, scientists have begun studying aloe for other potential medical benefits, including anti-tumor properties. NASA has already found a new, surprising use for this herb: It can clear formaldehyde from airtight rooms.

As with most herbs, however, what has most brought aloe back into the public eye is its commercial potential. In the 1970s, corporate marketers discovered that aloe could be used to treat everything from minor sunburn to more serious electrical burns and even burns from cancer radiation therapy. The plant has been popular ever since.

Expert consulted
Gail E. Wagner, Ph.D.
President of the Society for Economic Botany
Associate professor in the department
of anthropology
University of South Carolina
Columbia

Do not ingest the leaf. It can cause intense cramping and is a potentially toxic, habit-forming laxative. Aloe may delay deep wound healing, so do not use the gel on any surgical incision.

Angelica

Angelica archangelica
Also known as root of the Holy Ghost; herb of the angel

According to Renaissance folklore, God answered the prayers of a Benedictine monk by revealing angelica as a cure for the Great Plague. Today, this bitter herb appears in European patent medicines, including sedatives, digestive aids, and cramp relievers. Some herbalists believe that angelica promotes circulation and works on congestion, colds, flu, menstrual irregularities, and cramps.

Angelica has a bitter taste that appears to trigger a sensory response in the mouth that can aid digestion and ease gas and stomach cramps. Its roots and leaves are used as a tincture or a tea.

Be aware that angelica looks like hemlock, a deadly poison, so never harvest angelica in the wild. Also, use angelica sparingly and only for short periods of time, since prolonged use can cause rashes or sun sensitivity.

Astragalus

Astragalus membranaceous
Also known as huang qi; milk-vetch root

Used for more than 2,000 years by traditional Chinese healers, astragalus has also gained respect among Western herbalists since its effects as an immune-system booster came to light.

WOMAN TO WOMAN

She Restores Her Energy Level with Astragalus

Jennifer Reid, a naturopathic physician from Gresham, Oregon, ran herself into the ground by working for a law firm, pursuing a psychology degree, and training for triathlons—all at the same time. She became so sapped of energy that doctors didn't know what to make of it. Then, by chance, she stepped into an herbal store. That visit revitalized her in ways she never would have thought possible. Here is her story.

When I was in my early twenties (I'm now 34), I became sick. For almost two years, I could barely climb out of bed, and when I did, I'd get out of breath and become so weak that I couldn't stand up. This was especially frustrating because I was used to getting up super early, around 5:00 A.M., and then running 6 to 10 miles and pedaling 30 to 50 miles on my bike. Afterward, I'd shower and go to class. Later in the day, I'd work as a runner at a law firm. For a while, I was also going to paralegal school at night. I'd come home at 10:00 P.M., jump in the pool, and swim about a mile. I was so busy that I never cooked. I was nuts. No wonder I got chronic fatigue syndrome.

It started with the flu. I was so sick that I missed two weeks of work. I felt nauseated all the time, and my legs were shaky. Standing up and walking one step was a major ordeal. When I tried using the exercise bike, one minute of pedaling was about all I could take.

Different doctors tested me, first telling me that I had

Herbalists say that astragalus is a natural choice for anyone who might have a weakened immune system, from cold sufferers to cancer patients. Evidence indicates that astragalus helps the body produce protective antibodies and interferon as well as white blood cells. It also contains high amounts of a type of molecule that seems to have anti-cancer qualities. The healing properties are found in the root only.

Astragalus is sold in tincture, tonic, and cap-multiple sclerosis, then leukemia. I was also tested for Lyme disease and even AIDS. It was none of these. One doctor sent me to a psychologist because I was depressed. Of course I was; I couldn't exercise and I was frustrated. But depression was the effect, not the cause, of my condition. Finally, I decided to take my situation in hand and do my own detective work. I started reading medical abstracts and soon realized that what I had was chronic fatigue syndrome.

I immediately made some significant changes in my diet and mental outlook, hoping I could help myself to get better. But it took three months of slow recovery before I was able to walk downtown again.

It was during that walk that I saw an interesting herbal shop. I just went in to browse but soon found myself talking to the owner. He knew right away that I had chronic fatigue and suggested I try a Chinese medicine formula that had astragalus as the main ingredient. He told me how astragalus has good antiviral and antibacterial components. It also helps your immune system.

I began getting results almost immediately, and there were no side effects. Soon I was feeling really strong, like I'd had a great boost in my immune system. Since then, I've gotten married and recently had the healthiest little baby girl after the greatest pregnancy in the world. I definitely consider that visit to that herbal store to be the turning point in my recovery and my life—it motivated me to go back to school and earn a degree in naturopathy. It opened my eyes to how beneficial medicinal herbs can be.

sule form. Be patient. It may take a few weeks to show its effects. Astragalus is generally regarded as safe.

Basil

Ocimum basilicum
Also known as sweet basil

A native of India, basil was introduced into Europe during ancient times. In some cultures, basil is regarded as a love token. In others, it is associated with hatred and misfortune.

Now a standard herb in many American kitchens, basil is used medicinally to treat a wide range of conditions, including diarrhea, fever, and jet lag. It may also improve memory.

Basil contains many antiviral compounds. It helps to relieve depression as well.

The leaves contain the medicinal substances. Fresh leaves rubbed on insect bites take away the itch. As an essential oil, basil is used for nervous exhaustion and mental fatigue. As a tincture, it helps in relieving coughs and bronchitis.

Herbalists advise not taking large amounts of basil tea (several cups per day) for extended periods. Also, the essential oil may irritate the skin if used in a high concentration.

Bearberry

Arctostaphylos uva-ursi
Also known as uva-ursi; bear's grape; mountain box

Marco Polo heard about bearberry's medicinal potential during his journey through Asia. It's unclear if he took this herb back home, but by the thirteenth century, bearberry was considered an important medicinal herb in Europe. This ground cover was so named because its bright red berries attract bears.

Bearberry is used by herbalists to treat chronic bladder infections by means of an antiseptic contained in the leaves. The leaves also contain antibiotic substances as well as compounds that can help reduce pain in the urinary tract.

Bearberry can be taken as a tincture, as a tea, or in capsules. Herbalists recommend not taking bearberry for more than two weeks because its leaves contain tannin, a natural compound that can irritate the stomach. Also, don't use it if you have a kidney disease because the tannin can cause more damage.

Black Cohosh

Cimicifuga racemosa
Also known as black snakeroot; bugbane; rattleroot; rattleweed; squawroot

Derived from the Algonquian word meaning "knobby, rough roots," black cohosh was used by American herbal healers in the 1800s to treat conditions as varied as snakebite, smallpox, and hypochondria.

Today we know that black cohosh provides a host of nutrients as well as chemicals that help the body produce and use a variety of hormones. Its relaxing and hormone-balancing qualities make it an ideal choice among herbalists for treatment of rheumatoid arthritis, painful or delayed menstruation, menstrual cramps, and hot flashes during menopause.

Select black cohosh in tinctures, capsules, or decoctions that use its root and rhizome, which is a horizontal, underground stem. Don't use the herb for more than six months at a time.

Black Haw

Viburnum prunifolium
Also known as stag bush; sweet viburnum; American sloe

Found throughout the eastern and central United States, black haw gained a reputation for preventing miscarriages among early Native Americans and pioneers.

Modern herbalists recommend black haw to ease menstrual cramps, ease bleeding after childbirth, and tone down menopausal symptoms. This herb contains four key substances: an aspirin-like compound, a powerful uterine relaxant, a sedative, and steroidlike compounds that may assist the liver in producing hormones.

The bark from its roots, trunk, and branches is best used either boiled down (decocted) into a hot drink or taken as a tincture. People with a history of kidney stones should consult a physician before using black haw, since this herb contains substances that can cause kidney stones.

Blue Cohosh

Caulophyllum thalictroides
Also known as papoose root; squawroot

Blue cohosh is one of the oldest-known American herbal remedies. Introduced into medicine in the 1820s, it earned praise for its ability to promote menstruation and to encourage labor.

Blue cohosh contains a chemical that actively stimulates contractions of the uterus and promotes blood flow to the pelvis. Top herbalists regard blue cohosh as a great choice to help relieve menstrual cramps. This herb also has a reputation for easing rheumatic pain and soothing nervous coughs.

The root and rhizome of blue cohosh can be taken as a tincture, decoction, or in capsules. The berries are poisonous.

Burdock

Arctium lappa
Also known as beggar's-buttons; clotbur; fox's clote

Burdock possesses a 3,000-year-old reputation for purifying blood and boosting immunity. Seventeenth-century herbalist Nicholas Culpeper declared that burdock root worked wonderfully on bites by "serpents and mad dogs."

Weedy in appearance with fierce, tenacious burrs, herbalists use burdock to treat burns, kidney problems, rheumatism, and lung infections. The herb contains a compound that both boosts the immune system and shows antidiabetic properties. In addition, burdock's diuretic and mild laxative properties help remove toxins from your body, making it a choice for psoriasis, eczema, and acne treatment, according to herbal practitioners. Herbalists use the leaves, roots, and seeds of this herb.

Generally regarded as safe, burdock can be used in the form of a tea or tincture or taken in capsules. Its tender leaves can be served raw, steamed, or sautéed.

Calendula

Calendula officinalis
Also known as marybud; pot marigold; gold-bloom

During the Dark Ages, medieval healers advised women to concoct a calendula potion to choose the best suitor. They would mix calendula with honey and white wine and rub the blend all over themselves, believing that their future husbands would appear in a dream.

Today, we've left behind superstitious romantic rituals in favor of the practical healing properties that this common garden plant offers. Its orange flower tops and petals contain chemicals that can help reduce inflammation, fight infection, and heal stubborn wounds. Primarily an herb for skin problems, calendula also may show promise in treatments for herpes simplex outbreaks, certain flu viruses, and skin cancer.

Calendula is generally considered to be a safe

THE NAME GAME

Down in the fields of Texas, wild plants that the locals call milkweeds grow in abundance. But if you ask herbal educator and Texas native Ginger Webb to dig up information about milkweed, she won't be able to help you. "Everything here is called milkweed. Many different plants got called milkweed because they all have a milky sap inside. That name doesn't really tell me anything," Webb says.

Just as one name can be attached to many different plants, one plant can go by many different names. "Someone is talking about coneflower and another person is talking about snakeroot. They are both talking about echinacea," says Webb, the herbal education coordinator for the American Botanical Council in Austin, Texas.

The best way to be accurate when discussing herbs is to use their botanical names, Webb says. The botanical name is the scientific identification botanists give to plants. No two plants have the same botanical name, so you're guaranteed to get the right herb when you use its official moniker.

Even for the most popular herbs, it's wise to know their proper names. For instance, the widely known term *ginseng* is used to describe three different plants. Two types, *Panax ginseng* (Korean ginseng) and *Panax quinquefolium* (American ginseng), are related. But what people call Siberian ginseng—with the botanical name of *Eleutherococcus senticosus*—isn't a true species of ginseng at all. "Learning the botanical names helps so that when you look up information about a plant, you know you are not getting information about some other plant," Webb says.

---

herb. Forms include teas, tinctures, skin-care creams, and ointments.

Chamomile

Matricaria recutita
Also known as German chamomile

Nicknamed "ground apple" by the ancient Greeks because of its smell, chamomile was also called maythen by the Anglo-Saxons, who regarded it as one of the nine sacred herbs given to the world by the god Woden.

Chamomile has been healing people for more than 2,000 years. It counteracts irritation, soothes upset tummies, shields against ulcers, relaxes muscle spasms, and fights off bacterial and fungal invaders.

A member of the daisy family, it contains a complex collection of compounds that protect and heal the body. One of its chemicals mends torn tissues and heals ulcers. Another kills staphylococcus and streptococcus infections.

You can use this herb in a tea or in tinctures or essential oils. If you're allergic to ragweed, asters, and chrysanthemums, however, you're apt to be allergic to chamomile as well. Don't confuse German chamomile with Roman chamomile, which is used in shampoos and cosmetics.

Chasteberry

Vitex agnus-castus
Also known as vitex; monk's pepper

Through the ages, chasteberry was used to quell sexual passion. Ancient Athenian women sacrificed chasteberry to the goddess Ceres as a symbol of chastity. Nineteenth-century women used chasteberry syrup to "suppress the desires of Venus."

Today, this highly studied perennial flowering shrub appears to balance hormones during menstruation and menopause. Herbalists say it influences the pituitary gland to stem secretions of the hormone prolactin and allow for a normal menstrual cycle. Chasteberry is the choice for women who experience chronic premenstrual syndrome, menstrual cramps, and menstrual irregularities. It may also be used to aid the body to regain a natural balance after using birth control pills.

The berries are used in teas and tinctures. Be patient. This is a slow-acting herb, so take it

regularly for months to reap its benefits. Be aware that chasteberry may counteract the effectiveness of birth control pills.

Comfrey

Symphytum officinale
Also known as boneset; knitback; bruisewort; healing-herb

This herb has been healing wounds since at least the first century B.C. Greek physician Dioscorides proclaimed it as the first completely medicinal herb, unassociated with superstitious practices. Later, however, comfrey baths became popular before weddings to repair the hymen and "restore virginity."

Comfrey has a long history of use, and most of our knowledge comes from tradition. In the past, it has been used to reduce inflammation, stimulate the immune system, and ease asthma, ulcers, and lung ailments. Because of safety concerns, however, herbalists no longer recommend it for internal use.

The plant's roots and leaves are used externally—in ointments, poultices, and compresses. Use only dried comfrey, avoiding fresh, young leaves. Do not use on deep or infected wounds; comfrey seems to promote rapid surface healing, which can trap dirt or pus in underlying tissue.

Cramp Bark

Viburnum opulus
Also known as guelder rose; high cranberry; red, rose, or water elder

Birds avoid the bright red berries of the cramp bark bush because they're bitter, but Siberians distill the berries into a soul-warming brew. For more than 700 years, this herb has been prescribed by herbal practitioners to help prevent menstrual cramps, excessive bleeding during menopause, muscle cramps, and pelvic pain.

Nearly identical to black haw, cramp bark is an easy-to-grow shrub with showy white flowers. But cramp bark seems to be a stronger remedy for muscle pain than black haw. That's because cramp bark contains substances that calm the muscle spasms and relax the uterus, which may be how it reduces heavy menstrual bleeding.

The bark is the medicinal part of this herb and is generally regarded as safe.

Dandelion

Taraxacum officinale
Also known as goat's beard; wild chicory; pisseabed; dent de lion

Although today people throughout the world regard this yellow-flowered herb as a troublesome weed, it has been used as a medicinal plant since the times of ancient Greece. Its name probably came from the imagination of a fifteenth-century surgeon, who compared the shape of the leaves to a lion's tooth, or *dens leonis*.

Dandelion's leaves and roots are used as a diuretic and a liver stimulant. Its roots contain a detoxifier that cleans out various bodily poisons associated with constipation, joint inflammation, acne, fluid retention, and urinary disorders.

Dandelion contains several substances that combine to stimulate bile flow and aid in fat digestion.

Don't use dandelion root without medical approval if you have gallbladder disease.

WOMEN ASK WHY

Dandelion is a common weed. Why is it suddenly so revered as an herb and as a salad ingredient? Is it really safe to ingest this stuff?

Dandelion is possibly one of the most misunderstood and underappreciated plants on Earth. People spend a lot of time and money every year to poison, dig up, and wipe out this useful flower. Dandelion's transition from nuisance to revered herb and salad ingredient really isn't so sudden. In fact, it has been regarded throughout history as a great healer and food source. It wasn't until people began obsessing about perfect lawns that it gained its reputation as a weed.

You can safely eat every part of the dandelion. Toss the fresh, edible flowers and leaves into salads, or cook the leaves like spinach. A tea made from the root, either fresh or dried, is a good liver medicine. Dandelion flowers have even been used to make wine.

When harvesting dandelion on your own, choose flowers that lie at least 1,000 feet away from a roadway. Also, only use plants that you absolutely know are free of herbicides and pesticides. When you get home, wash the plants well under running water to remove any clinging dirt.

The leaves taste best in early spring, but you can continue to gather the youngest, most tender shoots of the plant throughout the summer. After soaking them, rinse thoroughly and toss with olive oil and lemon juice. If they're too bitter, mix them with lettuce at first, then add more dandelion leaves with each serving. You will gradually acquire a palate for this backyard delicacy.

Note: If you have gallbladder disease, do not take dandelion root without medical approval.

Expert consulted
Ellen Evert Hopman
Professional member of the American Herbalists Guild
Author of Tree Medicine, Tree Magic *and* A Druid's Herbal for the Sacred Earth
Amherst, Massachusetts

Dong Quai

Angelica sinensis
Also known as dang gui; Chinese angelica

Dong quai, one of the most popular of all Chinese herbs, appears in ancient Chinese medical books dating back to 400 B.C. Revered in Asia as a versatile aid for women's health, dong quai has found use in traditional Chinese medicine in treating allergies, arthritis, nervousness, and high blood pressure.

Herbalists say that dong quai relaxes the uterus, regulates menstruation, reduces hot flashes, reverses vaginal dryness, and clears eczema and psoriasis. Dong quai contains vitamins B_{12} and E and other active compounds, including ferulic acid, which ease menstrual cramps, muscle spasms, and other types of pain. It also contains folate and biotin. These vitamins, along with B_{12}, stimulate the creation and development of red blood cells in the bone marrow, which seems to treat a type of anemia associated with menstrual problems.

The herb's root is used in tinctures, teas, or capsules. Herbalists recommend that you stop taking dong quai one week before your menstrual period and resume taking it at the end of your period since it can increase blood loss.

Echinacea

Echinacea angustifolia; E. purpurea
Also known as purple coneflower; Kansas or Missouri snakeroot

Echinacea is the world's most researched herb. Its use goes back to the North American Plains Indians, who used it as a remedy more often than any other plant.

WOMAN TO WOMAN
She Found Psoriasis Relief

Doris I. Young, 65, a teacher at Widener University School of Nursing in Chester, Pennsylvania, has had the skin disease psoriasis since she was 10 years old. Her doctor recommended a powerful vitamin D drug, a cancer-treatment medicine, or steroids, but these options struck her as too severe, especially since she only has a moderate case. Because she grew up using herbs, she searched for a more natural means of treatment. She found one that works for her. Here's her story.

Psoriasis is a skin condition in which your cells reproduce too quickly in certain areas and so pile up faster than they can be shed. You know how skin sloughs off all the time? Well, my skin sloughs off at a faster rate. So I get these big flakes of skin, and these flakes itch. Because of the itch, I scratch and scratch, and I have all these scales. My skin also tightens up.

I've had to live with psoriasis, but it has been so bothersome. When I first looked into treatment, I was told about some really powerful medications. One was a vitamin D drug that was extremely expensive and couldn't guarantee results. Another was the cancer-treatment drug methotrexate, which slows down cell division.

Today, echinacea is America's most popular medicinal herb. It is used primarily for colds, flu, infections, slow-healing wounds, and overall immune-boosting.

Echinacea contains many biologically active substances, including some that strengthen the immune system and kill viruses.

The root is used medicinally in tinctures or capsules. Don't use echinacea if you have tuberculosis or an autoimmune condition such as leukosis (a precursor of leukemia), multiple sclerosis, lupus, or any collagen disease. Also, avoid using it if you're allergic to plants in the daisy family such as marigolds and chamomile.

What happens with cancer is that cells multiply too fast, just like with psoriasis. But anti-cancer medications have all those side effects, so I was not interested in that. If my psoriasis were worse, then I certainly would have considered them, but I'm not that bad. The drugs I have tried, such as corticosteroids, drove me crazy. I got fat, and I retained water. But what I hated most of all was that I couldn't think straight. I would never do that again.

Looking for alternatives, I learned that evening primrose oil is used in Great Britain for eczema, which is similar to psoriasis. As a nurse, I researched it first to confirm that it didn't interact with any other medications or supplements I take. After I started the evening primrose, I realized that my skin flakes were not as large as they used to be. The skin didn't seem to be reproducing as quickly. I itched less, and I didn't have that tight feeling. My skin still needed lubrication on the outside, but evening primrose oil seemed to lubricate it from the inside.

The great thing about evening primrose oil—and herbs in general—is that it has helped treat more than one condition. As a bonus, evening primrose has reduced my problems with asthma. In combination with other herbs, it has helped decrease my bronchial spasms. I also have high blood pressure, and evening primrose oil is thought to bring that down as well.

Eucalyptus

Eucalyptus globulus
Also known as blue gum; fever tree

In the land down under, eucalyptus trees engulf more than three-quarters of the continent. Aborigines and early Australian settlers quenched their thirst by drinking water stored in its roots. The tree was introduced to North America and Europe in the nineteenth century by the director of the Melbourne Botanical Gardens.

Eucalyptus leaves contain a chemical that herbalists think eases respiratory infections such as bronchitis, sore throats, coughs, fevers, and laryngitis. The aromatic oils of eucalyptus tea secrete through the lungs, where they loosen and remove mucus, which can then be cleared out by coughing.

Eucalyptus leaves are brewed into teas, and its essential oil appears in cough drops, nasal inhalers and sprays, sore-muscle rubs, and other preparations. Taking more than 4,000 milligrams a day can cause nausea, vomiting, and diarrhea. Do not use this herb if you have inflammatory disease of the bile ducts or severe liver disease. Do not use the essential oil for more than two weeks at a time or apply to the face. It may irritate the skin if used in a high concentration.

Evening Primrose

Oenothera biennis
Also known as tree primrose; scabbish; cure-all

The Iroquois Indians used evening primrose as a hemorrhoid remedy. The Cherokees drank evening primrose tea as a weight-loss tonic and applied the hot root externally for the treatment of hemorrhoids.

Today, both mainstream doctors and herbalists recommend using the oil extracted from the seeds of this nocturnally blossoming herb to ease a wide range of problems, some specific to women. Evening primrose oil helps to lessen some menopausal symptoms as well as chronic inflammatory conditions, such as eczema, hay fever, asthma, and arthritis. Its oil is abundant in essential fatty acids (EFAs), which help the body to manufacture substances that lower blood pressure, control stomach acids and body temperature, and regulate inflammation. It also shows promise as a fighter against America's top killers, heart disease and cancer.

THE HERBAL KITCHEN
Boosting Nutrition with Herbs

By adding a pinch of this or that to spice up your meals, you're doing more than enhancing the flavor of your meal. You're spicing up your overall health.

"Adding herbs to your cooking is a great way to boost nutrition. Many herbs are high in vitamins, minerals, and antioxidants," says Jennifer Reid, N.D., a naturopathic physician in Gresham, Oregon.

The bits of garlic clove swimming in your pasta sauce act as a natural antibiotic against infections and help to lower blood pressure and cholesterol. Basil adds flavor to a homemade pizza, but it also improves digestion and mental stimulation.

"Basically, every cooking spice can be considered a good digestive herb that also fights bacteria," says Mindy Green, a founding and professional member of the American Herbalists Guild, director of educational services for the Herb Research Foundation in Boulder, Colorado, and coauthor of *Aromatherapy: A Complete Guide to the Healing Art.* "But each herb has its own personality and requires its own special preparation."

If you follow these ground rules, you'll reap maximum health benefits from edible herbs.

Keep a lid on. An herb's volatile oils, which contain many of its healing properties, can escape into the air if they're left to boil in a pot without a lid, says Green.

Activate astragalus. This is one herb that must always be cooked for you to benefit from its immune-boosting and cold-fighting powers. "Even if you bought fresh astragalus and infused it in tea or juice, you're not going to get the same benefits you would if you had cooked it," says Green.

Don't skip supplements. Edible herbs lack the full nutritional clout that herbal supplements provide. "If you were adding herbs for their medicinal effect, you'd need to take quite a bit to reach a therapeutic dose," says Dr. Reid. "Adding sage to a stew will add flavor, but it will probably not have a noticeable effect on drying up a cold. Taking sage capsules would be much more effective."

Evening primrose oil is usually taken in capsule form and is generally regarded as safe.

Fennel

Foeniculum vulgare
Also known as sweet fennel

Ancient Romans believed that serpents sucked the juice of fennel to improve their eyesight. Ancient Greeks regarded fennel as an aid to weight loss. In medieval times, church-goers chewed fennel seeds to subdue stomach rumblings.

Rich in volatile oils, fennel seeds taste faintly of licorice and are often used to flavor pickles, candies, and breads. Medicinally, the seeds and the fresh stems and bulbs are used to relieve flatulence, aid digestion, regulate appetite, fight infection, heal snakebites, and increase the flow of milk in nursing mothers. Fennel seems to work in the digestive system by soothing the small and large intestines.

Add fennel seeds to food or brew them into teas. Fennel tinctures and capsules are also available. Don't use them medicinally for more than six weeks, however, without supervision by a health care practitioner qualified in herbal remedies.

Feverfew

Chrysanthemum parthenium;
Tanacetum parthenium
Also known as featherfew; flirtwort; vetter-voo

Seventeenth-century herbalists recommended feverfew as a good herb for getting rid of bad headaches. In the past, women took feverfew to stimulate the expulsion of the placenta after birth and to resolve a host of uterine disorders.

Today, the leaves are used to reduce swelling, relax blood vessels, aid digestion, promote menstruation, and stop headaches. Feverfew may stop throbbing headaches, including migraines, by inhibiting hormones that help to constrict blood vessels. Daily use may help prevent migraines from starting. Scientists theorize that feverfew's active compounds hinder inflammation-inducing agents in the body.

You can chew fresh feverfew leaves or add them to salads. You can infuse them into vinegar or oil as well. Feverfew can also be brewed into a tea or taken freeze-dried in capsules. The capsules must contain at least 0.2 percent parthenolide to be effective. Fresh feverfew leaves can cause mouth sores in sensitive people. Also, avoid using it if you're taking blood-thinning medicines, because feverfew can affect clotting rates.

Garlic

Allium sativum

Also known as stinking rose

This humble gray bulb was, and still is, used worldwide by all three classic healing systems: traditional Chinese medicine, traditional European medicine, and Ayurveda. In the first century B.C., Greek physician Dioscorides declared

---

GARLIC AND BAD BREATH

There's a reason that garlic's nickname is "stinking rose," and we all know what it is. It's the same reason people avoid standing too close while talking with us after we've eaten a pizza that has been spiced with the stuff. Fresh garlic contains sulfur compounds, which deliver that pungent, rotten egg odor, explains Jennifer Reid, N.D., a naturopathic physician in Gresham, Oregon.

Among medicinal herbs, garlic has been revered for centuries by Greek and Roman healers. In the past two decades, more than 1,000 research studies have been published about garlic's role as a natural antibiotic, bacteria fighter, and cholesterol reducer. Specifically, its sulfur-scented healing compound, called allicin, is activated whenever garlic cloves are crushed, cut, or chewed. Allicin is also released when enteric-coated garlic products, such as capsules, are broken down in the intestines.

So if you love garlic, what can you do to camouflage its odor? You could convince your close friends to eat garlic with you. Or you could end a garlic-laden meal by nibbling a sprig of parsley. Fresh parsley sprigs contain a high level of chlorophyll, and chlorophyll is the key ingredient in many breath fresheners, explains Dr. Reid.

You can also prevent bad breath by taking enteric-coated garlic products or organic odorless garlic powder capsules in lieu of the clove itself, but garlic's stubborn odor will permeate through your skin whenever you sweat, says Dr. Reid.

---

that garlic "clears the arteries and opens the mouths of the veins"—a fact supported by science today.

Garlic helps lower blood cholesterol and blood pressure, prevent blood clots, and improve the overall health of the cardiovascular system. The medicinal source can be found inside garlic cloves, where a sulfur-containing amino acid called alliin resides. When garlic is crushed, alliin converts into allicin, a potent but unstable antibiotic. In addition to its cardiovascular benefits, garlic also combats bacterial and fungal infections. Further, studies suggest that it may help to prevent cancer.

To enjoy the full healing power of garlic, experts advise that you eat raw cloves, but you can also cook it, drink it as a maceration (steeped in water or milk overnight), or swallow garlic capsules. You shouldn't use garlic supplements if you're on anticoagulants because garlic can thin your blood and increase bleeding. For the same reasons, don't use garlic before surgery. And don't use it if you're taking hypoglycemic drugs. Finally, avoid using fresh garlic while nursing, since it may give the baby gas or indigestion.

Ginger

Zingiber officinale
Also known as Jamaican ginger; African ginger; Cochin ginger

Emperor Shen Nung immortalized ginger's healing powers in the *Pen Tsao Ching (The Classic Book of Herbs)* in 3000 B.C., and it is still widely used in China today.

Ginger surpasses all other herbs when it comes to suppressing the queasiness of motion sickness, and studies show that it also works better than the active ingredient in over-the-counter drugs like Dramamine. Ginger settles upset stomachs, relieves vomiting, and eases gas pain and diarrhea by stimulating saliva flow and digestive activity. Its gingerols and shogaols are considered effective antinausea workhorses.

Take fresh or dried gingerroot in teas, tinctures, or capsules, or add it to food dishes. Since ginger may increase bile secretion, anyone with gallstones should check with a health care practitioner qualified in herbal remedies before using the dried root in therapeutic amounts.

Avoid it if you have ulcers, since it will overstimulate the stomach, herbalists say.

Ginkgo

Ginkgo biloba
Also known as maidenhair tree

The seeds of the ginkgo tree have been used as both food and medicine for thousands of years, but today, we use the leaves of the plant.

Ginkgo is considered a good anti-aging herb because it benefits organs usually diminished by time: the eyes, brain, blood vessels, and cardiovascular system. Scientists have learned that concentrated ginkgolide, a substance extracted from the leaves, sharpens memory, boosts concentration, reduces anxiety, lessens the symptoms of Alzheimer's disease, lowers blood pressure, relieves headaches, and improves a litany of circulation problems.

Ginkgo also contains derivatives of a compound called terpene, which acts as a bodyguard for the brain, protecting against blood clots and nerve damage. Ginkgo's flavonoids help stop the action of damaging free radicals.

Purchase ginkgo extracts that contain standardized amounts of ginkgolide for maximum benefits. Experts suggest products whose labels say "24/6," which means the product contains 24 percent glycosides and 6 percent terpenes. Diarrhea, vomiting, and dermatitis may occur if you take more than 240 milligrams of concentrated ginkgo daily. The usual daily dose is 120 milligrams.

Avoid taking ginkgo with antidepressant MAO inhibitor drugs such as phenelzine sulfate (Nardil) or tranylcypromine (Parnate), aspirin or other nonsteroidal anti-inflammatory medications, or blood-thinning medications such as warfarin (Coumadin).

Ginseng

Panax ginseng (Korean ginseng); P. quinquefolium (American ginseng)

Also known as sang; root of life; a dose of immortality

For thousands of years, ginseng has had a nearly mythical reputation as a cure-all herb. Explorer Marco Polo wrote of this prized wonder drug, and Native Americans used American ginseng, hoping it would help with menstrual problems, headaches, exhaustion, fever, colic, vomiting, and earaches. Today, many Asians use ginseng to renew and enhance sexual desire and ease difficult childbirth.

Another kind of ginseng, Siberian (*Eleutherococcus senticosus*), is not a true form of ginseng, but it shares certain properties with the Korean and American herbs.

Science hasn't completely proven that ginseng helps with all of those conditions, but scientists have discovered that the root contains at least 18 different hormonelike substances. These fight stress and fatigue, protect the liver, and prevent memory loss. This herb is often used to relieve stress-related hot flashes at menopause.

The root can be chewed or made into a tea. Ginseng is also available in capsules, tablets, and liquid extracts. Avoid it while consuming caffeine or other stimulants because it may cause irritability. Don't take it if you have high blood pressure.

WOMEN ASK WHY

If ginkgo is so good for my memory, why do I keep forgetting to take it?

If you forget to take your daily ginkgo capsules or tincture drops, chances are you're also forgetting other things. Car keys lost—again? Forget to buy milk at the supermarket?

To get the best results from taking ginkgo, I recommend that a woman first determine the cause of her forgetfulness. Inadequate sleep and lack of regular exercise can contribute to fuzzy memory. So can a poor diet, everyday stress, and simply growing older. She needs to practice healthy eating and living habits. That means eating meals low in fat and sugar, and rich in fruits, vegetables, and grains. If you also get a minimum of seven hours of sleep each night and exercise for 30 minutes at least three times each week, you'll maximize the many benefits ginkgo offers.

In addition to ranking as the top herb for boosting memory, ginkgo is also great for improving circulation to the legs and delivering oxygen to the brain.

I recommend taking ginkgo every morning so that it works all day long. If you take it at night, you're apt to remember your dreams better than your daytime activities. To remember to take ginkgo every morning, put it where you're bound to see it. You might try keeping the jar next to a glass on the kitchen counter next to the sink. Or you could place it and a glass next to your toothbrush in the bathroom. You could even stow it with your car keys, so you don't head out the door without either.

Once you get into the ginkgo-taking habit, you'll be amazed at what other things you remember. And you'll probably always have those car keys at your fingertips.

Expert consulted
Kathi Keville
Author of Herbs for Health and Healing
Director of the American Herb Association
Nevada City, California

Goldenseal

Hydrastis canadensis
Also known as orange root; yellow root; jaundice root; eye balm

Native to North America, goldenseal was used extensively by Native Americans as a clothing dye and a war paint as well as a remedy. The wrinkled, chrome-yellow root was used by the Cherokee to soothe inflammation and spark appetite. The Iroquois washed sore eyes with it. The Micmac applied goldenseal to chapped lips.

Although goldenseal is the third best-selling herb in the United States, there has been little scientific study of its usefulness. Nevertheless, many herbalists depend on goldenseal to alleviate sinus infections, colds and flu, laryngitis, sore throats, mouth sores, colitis, gastritis, earaches, and vaginal infections. Goldenseal root contains substances that act as natural antibiotics, inflammation stoppers, uterine tonics, and digestive helpers.

Herbalists use the roots in teas, tinctures, capsules, eyewashes, gargles, ear drops, douches, and disinfectant salves. Goldenseal is safe when used topically, but do not use it internally for more than three weeks, since it may irritate your mucous membranes. Also, don't use goldenseal if you have high blood pressure.

Green Tea

Camellia sinensis
Also known, in China, as cha

Green tea has been used in China for more than 5,000 years, and it has become so common in our own culture that you may overlook its important role as a medicinal herb.

Green tea is amazingly versatile. It contains polyphenols, or catechins, that protect your heart by lowering cholesterol levels and improving the way your body metabolizes fats. These substances also fight bacterial invaders. They may help guard against cancer by collecting free radicals that can damage cells and push them toward uncontrolled growth. Green tea contains fluoride, so it can lessen the risk of tooth decay. It is also used to treat insect bites.

People with asthma benefit from drinking green tea because it contains a substance, a close cousin of caffeine, that opens up bronchial tubes.

Green tea leaves are primarily brewed to drink, but you can also use them to make an effective poultice or compress.

Women with irregular heartbeats should limit their intake to no more than two cups of green tea daily because the caffeinelike alkaloids can speed up heart rates. Its bitter taste stimulates gastric acid production, so green tea should be consumed in limited amounts by people with stomach ulcers.

Hawthorn

Crataegus oxycantha;
C. laevigata; C. monogyna
Also known as May blossom;
whitethorn; haw

In the past, this fast-growing hedge and ornamental shrub had been used for weak stomachs, edema, and as a first-aid tool to draw splinters. By the turn of this century, however, herbal doctors began prescribing hawthorn for cardiac weakness, heart pain, and irregular heartbeats.

Now, hawthorn's red berries, white flowers, and leaves are recognized by herbalists as useful for long-term cardiovascular health. They contain compounds that dilate arteries and lower blood pressure, when taken for at least six months. Hawthorn also stimulates circulation and helps deliver oxygen to the heart.

THE HERBAL KITCHEN
Immune-Enhancing Herbal Soup

Whether you're looking to stop a cold in its tracks or fend off the flu, or just searching for a fortifying soup to banish sluggish, achy, or stressed-out feelings, try this easy soup recipe. Bolstered with helping herbs, it is offered by herbalist Rosemary Gladstar, director of the Sage Mountain Herbal Education Center in East Barre, Vermont, and author of *Herbal Healing for Women*.

- 2 16-ounce cans of chicken soup (or 32 ounces of miso soup for vegetarians)
- ¾ cup water
- 1 small red onion, diced
- 1 small red pepper, sliced thin
- 1 teaspoon lemon juice
- 2 cloves garlic, minced
- 1 slice fresh astragalus
- 1 tablespoon burdock root (fresh or dried)
- 1 tablespoon dandelion root (fresh or dried)
- 1 tablespoon Siberian ginseng (dried)
- ¼ teaspoon thyme (fresh or dried)
- 2 pinches cayenne pepper

Pour the chicken soup into a 3-quart pot. Stir in the water, onion, red pepper, lemon juice, garlic, astragalus, burdock root, dandelion root, ginseng, thyme, and cayenne pepper. If using fresh burdock root and dandelion slices, mix them directly into the soup. If using dried burdock root and dandelion, place these herbs in a mesh bag and then put it into the pot. Cover the pot and simmer for 15 minutes. Remove the astragalus slice and mesh bag (if you've used it) before serving. The chicken flavoring may overpower the taste of these medicinal herbs, but be assured that they will help fortify your immune system against invading germs and energy-draining stress.

Hawthorn is primarily taken as a tea but may also be used as a tincture. Have your doctor monitor your heart health if you take hawthorn regularly for more than three weeks. In some instances, you may need lower doses of other medicines, such as drugs for high blood pressure. If you have heart valve problems that cause low blood pressure, don't use hawthorn without a physician's supervision.

Kava Kava

Piper methysticum
Also known as intoxicating pepper

Native to tropical forests, kava kava is a staple at some Polynesian religious rites, during which participants drink it as a fermented liquor. Kava kava can relax you and evoke restful sleep without numbing your mind or leaving you with a hangover.

Kava kava belongs to a class of herbs called nervines, which seem to nudge into action the part of our nervous systems that helps us to relax. It is effective against tension headaches, anxiety, insomnia, and cramps caused by endometriosis. The dried root of kava kava reduces muscle spasms, soothes pain, and heightens your sense of well-being.

Sometimes used as a tea, kava kava is also available in tinctures and capsules. Do not exceed the recommended doses. Because the herb is a mild sedative and muscle relaxant, never take it with alcohol or barbiturates, and use caution when driving or operating equipment.

Lady's-Mantle

Alchemilla vulgaris
Also known as ladies mantle; lion's foot; bear's foot

Highly astringent and rich in tannins, lady's-mantle was used to heal wounds sustained in battle during the fifteenth and sixteenth centuries. As its name implies, this herb with gray-green leaves and lacy blooms is considered a valuable gynecological remedy as well.

Its astringent properties make it an excellent herb for normalizing bleeding from heavy periods or fibroid tumors. It also improves uterine tone, subdues menopausal hot flashes, and soothes mild menstrual aches and pains.

In addition, its leaves and flowers help close and heal wounds. When they're taken internally, they help relieve bleeding and diarrhea.

Use the leaves, stems, and flowers of lady's-mantle internally in a tea or tincture, or externally as an herbal wash or poultice. The herb is generally considered safe.

Lavender

Lavandula officinalis; L. angustifolia; L. vera
Also known as true lavender; garden lavender

Ancient Greeks imported lavender from Syria because of its fragrance, which freshened rooms, perfumes, and baths.

Today, lavender is a key ingredient in smelling salts.

The fragrant, volatile oil in its blossoms contains more than 100 chemical compounds that calm the central nervous system. As a tea, it tastes soapy, so you may want to add honey. Lavender is also taken as a tincture or used externally as an essential oil in baths, facial steams, and massage oils. It is generally considered to be safe.

Lemon Balm

Melissa officinalis
Also known as sweet balm; balm; melissa

Linked since ancient times with bees, lemon balm's botanical name, *Melissa*, comes from the Greek word for "honeybee." Up until the eighteenth century, lemon balm was thought to renew youth.

Today, its fuzzy, citrus-scented leaves are used to calm tension, raise the spirits, and relieve depression, insomnia, nervousness, and tension headaches. Since it relieves gas, it can tame digestive discomfort, especially when stress is the cause. It contains oils that are full of terpenes, substances that have antiviral properties and may help to fight herpes outbreaks. Women also rely on lemon balm to relax uterine spasms that cause painful periods.

Lemon balm is usually taken as a tea or used in ointments or as a calming bath. It's considered to be a safe herb.

Licorice

Glycyrrhiza glabra
Also known as sweet wood

Used as medicine for more than 2,500 years and nicknamed the "great detoxifier" in China, licorice is thought to drive poisons from the body. In seventeenth-century England, licorice was boiled with figs to silence coughs and chest pains.

The root of this versatile herb, sometimes called the grandfather of herbs, is found in many herbal formulas for women because it contains estrogen-like compounds. This makes it valuable for regulating hormones at menopause. In addition, licorice also contains a compound called glycyrrhizin, which is 50 times sweeter than sugar. It also has substances that help fight inflammation, allergies, and arthritis.

To treat arthritis and allergic conditions, use it in a tincture; for asthma and bronchitis, take it in a syrup, herbalists recommend. For ulcers,

WOMEN ASK WHY

I love licorice! Can eating licorice candy really help my cough or sore throat go away?

That flexible candy stick you love munching on at the movie theater shares its name and sweet taste with the medicinal plant, but nothing else. Licorice candy contains mostly corn syrup, sugar, and artificial flavoring. The medicinal herb form of licorice contains glycyrrhizin, a bacteria-killing, nonsugar sweetener.

Licorice is well-regarded among herbalists for its versatility in treating many conditions. Licorice tea soothes the mucous membranes, making it a preferred choice for coughs, asthma, and sore throats. For the best medicinal form, select deglycyrrhizinated licorice extracts (DGLE).

If you enjoy licorice candy but want medicinal benefits, too, try the fresh (and genuine) licorice sticks available in health food stores. You'll enjoy their sweet taste, and they may clear up any congestion that has you down.

Keep in mind that ingesting excessive amounts of licorice can cause water retention, headaches, or high blood pressure from potassium loss. Do not use licorice for more than four to six weeks, and avoid it if you have diabetes, high blood pressure, or a heart, liver, or kidney condition.

Expert consulted
Rosita Arvigo
Master herbalist and doctor of naprapathy
*   (a form of chiropractic)*
Author of Rainforest Remedies
Director of the Ix Chel Tropical Research
*   Foundation*
Belize, Central America

drink it as a decoction to reduce stomach acid. Never use licorice if you have diabetes, high blood pressure, liver or kidney disorders, or low potassium levels, or for more than four to six weeks.

Marshmallow

Althaea officinalis
Also known as cheeses

Marshmallow's slippery, sweet main ingredient was used for thousands of years as a soothing cure for coughs, sore throats, wheezing, and irritated skin. It gained a reputation as a tasty treat only a few centuries ago, when a spongy mix of sugar, egg whites, and ground marshmallow root, called *pate de guimauve*, became a trendy royal dessert in Europe. Unfortunately, modern-day marshmallow candy lacks any real marshmallow root.

Researchers have discovered why this pretty marsh-dwelling plant heals wounded skin and soothes mucous membranes. The root contains high amounts of a slippery, indigestible complex sugar, called mucilage, that coats, cools, and moisturizes wounded, inflamed tissues from the throat to the intestines to the urinary tract. Herbalists also use marshmallow root for mouth sores, gastritis, peptic ulcers, irritating coughs, varicose veins, and burns.

Take marshmallow as a cold or hot tea, or use it as a poultice of mashed roots. Because it will coat the linings of your digestive tract, keep in mind that marshmallow may slow absorption of other medications taken at the same time.

Milk Thistle

Silybum marianum
Also known as Mary thistle; Marian thistle; lady's thistle

The famous English herbalist known only as Gerald described milk thistle as "the best remedy that grows, against all melancholy diseases." In the Middle Ages, melancholy was associated with any liver- or bile-related illness.

Herbalists recommend this herb's seeds for increasing the secretion and flow of bile from the liver and gallbladder. Milk thistle's active ingredient, silymarin, is one of the strongest liver protectors known. Scientists have learned that the compound improves cirrhosis, hepatitis, and liver damage caused by toxic chemicals. As an antioxidant, it may be 10 times stronger than vitamin E.

Take milk thistle in tea, capsules, tablets, and tinctures. It's considered to be a safe herb.

Motherwort

Leonurus cardiaca
Also known as mother herb; heart heal; lion's tail; lion's ear

Motherwort was once regarded as a powerful defender against wicked spirits, and it was used for thousands of years to dispel doldrums and anxiety. The ancient Chinese believed motherwort could lengthen life. In the past, its dull green leaves and purplish blooms were called upon to induce menstruation and alleviate fainting.

Motherwort's leaves and flowers contain substances that promote menstrual bleeding. It also contains mild sedatives and relaxants that may temporarily lower blood pressure. Herbalists believe these compounds soothe the stress of premenstrual tension and menopausal hot flashes, restore cardiac health, and tone down a rapid heartbeat brought on by anxiety.

Use motherwort as a tea or tincture. For tension relief, it may take about 15 minutes before you feel the effects. It is generally regarded as safe.

Mullein

Verbascum thapsus
Also known as candlewick; velvet dock; Arron's rod; Peter's staff

Mullein's tall stems, which are covered in fine down, were once burned as tapers in funeral processions. Greek physician Dioscorides used the herb for scorpion stings, eye problems, and toothaches.

Today herbalists use mullein's velvety leaves and flowers to help treat bronchitis, colds and flu, coughs, earaches, emphysema, and laryngitis. It works for respiratory complaints because it helps bring up sticky phlegm, soothes sore throats, fights bacterial invaders, and stops muscle spasms that trigger coughs. It also contains compounds that inhibit flu viruses.

Use mullein in teas, tinctures, mouthwashes, and syrups. It is generally regarded as safe.

Nettle

Urtica dioica
**Also known as stinging nettle; wild
spinach**

Historically, Europeans used nettle gargles to ease sore, swollen throats and prepared nettle drinks to expel kidney stones by increasing urination. Native Americans used nettle to treat ills as varied as coughs, colds, epilepsy, gout, stomachaches, insanity, and even hair loss. Nineteenth-century Americans used nettle tea to treat diarrhea, dysentery, and hemorrhoids.

Today's herbalists are more judicious and realistic. They use nettle as a diuretic as well as an astringent to stop nosebleeds, wound bleeding, and heavy menstrual flow. Some herbalists believe it may also alleviate sinus problems, allergies, and hay fever. Used externally, nettle soothes insect bites and stings as well as burns.

WOMAN TO WOMAN
Taming the Symptoms of Menopause

Margit Echols, a 55-year-old Washington, New Jersey, quilt maker, wanted to take a natural approach to meeting the challenges of her menopause, which included hot flashes, feelings of anxiety, and interrupted sleep. She credits an herbal formula based on motherwort for keeping her hormones in balance and her symptoms subdued.

For about a year and a half, menopause really rocked my boat. I'd wake up sweating, and I'd go to the bathroom three or four times every night. During the day, the hot flashes were pretty severe, and I usually got anxious right before they hit. It was always this "uh-oh, here they come" sensation, and I'd feel all shaken up inside, and the sweat would start pouring out.

I truly believe in natural alternative medicines. That's why I didn't go to a conventional doctor for 25 years, except for my regular gynecological visits. I believe medicinal herbs are the best discovery I ever made. But I also know I can't just walk into a health food store and start buying herbs off the shelf. So I did nothing.

Then I met Kerry Adams, who's a practicing herbalist in my area. She and I worked on my menopause together. She tailors her practice to meet the individual needs of each woman she sees. For me, that meant an herbal tonic with nine herbs, with motherwort being one of the prominent ones. It was wonderful. Within two weeks of taking this tonic, my menopausal symptoms started quieting down. I now keep a supply of motherwort tea in the refrigerator and drink it whenever I feel hot flashes or night sweats coming on. Motherwort helps with my sleep, too, so I wake up feeling rested. It's not very pleasant-tasting, but it really works.

I believe nature has given us everything we need. We just have to learn how to see what she offers us and use it wisely. That's why I'm glad I found Kerry and motherwort.

Take this herb as a tea, tincture, or freeze-dried in capsules. It can also be used as a compress. Some people's allergy symptoms may worsen, rather than improve, after using nettle,

HERB AND DRUG INTERACTIONS

Even though herbs can be safer than over-the-counter drugs or prescriptions, they should be regarded as medicine. Don't take herbs and over-the-counter medications at the same time for the same condition, and inform your doctor of any herbs you take, especially if you're taking prescription medicines.

Not all herb-drug interactions are known. This table offers some potential interactions between herbs and medications for common conditions, based on medical research.

Type of Drug	Type of Herb	Possible Effects If Combined
Antidepressant drugs such as fluoxetine (Prozac), amitriptyline (Elavil), and imipramine (Trofranil)	Sedative herbs such as skullcap, passionflower, and valerian	Sedative side effects of the drug may increase.
Anti-allergy drugs such as diphenhydramine (Benadryl), hydroxyzine (Vistaril), and astemizole (Hismanal)	Sedative herbs such as skullcap, passionflower, and valerian	Drowsiness caused by antihistamine drugs may increase.
Blood pressure medicine such as enalapril (Vaseretic) and prazosin (Minizide)	Herbs with ingredients that may raise blood pressure, such as licorice	The drug's effects may lessen.
	Diuretic herbs and herbs with ingredients that may lower blood pressure, such as garlic and hawthorn	The drug's effects may be increased or altered.
Cardiac glycosides, which include digitalis medications, such as digoxin (Lanoxin)	Herbs with ingredients that can affect the cardiovascular system, such as coltsfoot, motherwort, hawthorn, and goldenseal	The drug's effects may increase.
Diuretics, such as furosemide (Lasix) and indapamide (Lozol)	Diuretic herbs such as dandelion, uva-ursi, buchu, and cornsilk	Diuretic effects may be much stronger, with a risk of abnormally low potassium levels.
Hypnotic and mild sedative drugs, such as diazepam (Valium), flurazepam, and alprazolam (Xanax)	Sedative herbs such as skullcap, passionflower, and valerian	The drug's sedative effect may increase.
Laxative drugs, such as docusate sodium (Colace) and psyllium (Metamucil), and polycarbophil (FiberCon)	Laxative herbs such as aloe, cascara sagrada, plantain, rhubarb, senna, and yellow dock	The drug's effects may increase.

so medical experts advise taking no more than one dose a day for the first few days.

Oatstraw

Avena sativa
Also known as wild oats

Oats have been cultivated as a food since at least 100 B.C. Its straw, made into a tea, was used as a folk remedy for nervous exhaustion and sleeplessness. Traditionally, a good soak in an oatstraw bath was said to relieve arthritis and rheumatism.

Today, oatstraw is considered an excellent tonic for the whole system. It treats tension headaches, insomnia, nervous exhaustion, and physical fatigue. Oatstraw contains calcium and silicic acid (a component of silica), reportedly making this herb a good tonic for hair, nails, and bones.

Its stems, leaves, and husks are used in teas and tinctures or as a healing wash for skin conditions. Oatstraw contains the grain protein gluten, so don't ingest it if you have gluten intolerance (celiac disease).

Partridgeberry

Mitchella repens
Also known as squaw vine; deer berry; mountain tea; winter clover; hive vine

From the Cherokee to the Iroquois, Native American women turned to this low-growing herb to alleviate menstrual cramps and soothe sore nipples while nursing.

Today this evergreen with shiny leaves and brilliant red berries is still considered among the best remedies for bringing on missed menstrual periods, easing cramps, and lightening heavy menstrual flow.

The leaves, stems, and berries are used in teas and tinctures. Partridgeberry is generally considered safe.

Passionflower

Passiflora incarnata
Also known as maypop; passion-vine; Holy Trinity flower

The exotic and intricate flowers of this plant reminded Spanish explorers and missionaries of the crown of thorns of Christ's passion—the crucifixion. Hence its name, which refers to spiritual suffering, not sexual passion.

Passionflower grows wild in the southern United States. Its flower, leaves, and vine contain sedatives, so it's used as a remedy for rattled nerves and for inducing sleep when anxiety or the insomnia of menopause interrupts nighttime rest. It may also help calm other conditions, such as hot flashes, abdominal pain, headaches, and high blood pressure, when they're related to stress.

Passionflower is usually taken as a tea or tincture. It's generally regarded as safe.

Peppermint

Mentha piperita
Also known as field mint

Across the globe and throughout the centuries, peppermint has earned a reputation as a stomach-soothing, gas-repressing, nausea-reversing herb. In medieval Europe, after-dinner peppermint jellies aided in digestion. Arabs finished dinners with a mint tea. The Cherokee used peppermint to treat vomiting, colic, and gas.

Today, peppermint's stature among herbalists as a medicinal herb to treat nausea, vomiting, indigestion, flatulence, hiccups, and stomach muscle spasms remains unchallenged. Peppermint leaves contain menthol-rich volatile oils, which act as a mild anesthetic to the stomach wall. They also contain tannins and bitters, which may kill many kinds of microorganisms and boost mental alertness. Peppermint eases anxiety and tension as well.

If using fresh peppermint, crush the leaves first. Otherwise, take this herb as a tea or tincture. It's generally regarded as a safe herb.

Red Clover

Trifolium pratense
Also known as purple clover; meadow trefoil

Long, long ago, red clover was used strictly as fodder crop for cattle. Then, in medieval times, Christians associated this three-leafed grass with the Trinity. The Chinese relied on red clover's sap as a remedy for colds and influenza. Native Americans used the herb to treat menopausal symptoms.

Red clover blossoms contain estrogen-like substances that can help make your menstrual cycle more regular, enhance fertility, and balance hormones at menopause. Its flowers also contain calcium, magnesium, potassium, and vitamins B and C. They're used internally as a cleanser for skin complaints as well as a medicine for coughs and bronchitis.

This herb is primarily used in teas, tinctures, and compresses.

Rosemary

Rosmarinus officinalis
Also known as incensier

A symbol for remembrance, rosemary is a Mediterranean native shrub that was reputedly first grown in England in the fourteenth century by Philippa of Hainault, wife of Edward III.

A relative of mint, rosemary is an ideal choice to counter exhaustion, weakness, jet lag, and breast pain. Herbalists think that rosemary may help ease breast pain by acting as a drying agent to fluid-filled cysts. Plus, it helps balance out-of-whack hormones. According to herbalists, it's fortified with more than a dozen antioxidants, which mop up free radicals and help prevent aging in cells. It also contains a half-dozen compounds that reportedly prevent the breakdown of a brain chemical that plays a vital role in cognition and reasoning. People with Alzheimer's disease often have a deficit of this chemical.

Rosemary essential oil is also popular among aromatherapists for treating mild depression. It contains a compound that is believed to stimulate the central nervous system.

The leaves and stems are used in teas, tinctures, and essential oils. Rosemary may cause excessive menstrual bleeding. Avoid rosemary essential oil if you have epilepsy or hypertension.

St. John's Wort

Hypericum perforatum
Also known as hypericum; St.-Joan's-wort

Known as a wound healer since 500 B.C., this medicinal herb was gathered and burned annually by European peasants on June 24, St. John's Day, to stave off goblins and devils. Its yellow flowers, which release crimson juice when crushed, became a symbol of the blood of St. John the Baptist.

This weedy-looking herb contains at least three key medicinal substances. One of them, hypericin, protects the brain's serotonin, the feel-good chemical. Taken internally, St. John's wort delivers a sedative and pain-reducing effect, making it an ideal choice among herbal healers to treat depression, anxiety, and tension. As a lotion, it helps heal bruises, varicose veins, and sunburn, possibly because it's an anti-inflamma-

tory. When using it for depression, make sure you buy St. John's wort that contains standardized levels of hypericin—0.3 percent—for best results. It may take two to six weeks to take effect.

You can use the leaves, stems, and flowers in tea, tincture, powder, capsules, tablets, and (for external use) oil. Be aware that this herb may cause sun sensitivity. Also, avoid taking it with other antidepressants unless you have your doctor's approval.

Skullcap

Scutellaria laterifolia
Also known as mad-dog weed; helmet flower

First used by Native Americans for rabies and menstrual problems, this herb, with its dish-shaped seedpods and delicate blue flowers, is now well-respected as a tonic that nourishes and revitalizes the nervous system.

Skullcap contains minerals (including calcium, iron, potassium, and magnesium) that help you deal with stress, tension headaches, anxiety, exhaustion, and depression. A mild "lullaby herb," skullcap promotes sound sleep without leaving you feeling groggy in the morning. It also eases the moodiness of premenstrual syndrome and severe mood changes during menopause.

Use skullcap's leaves and flowers in teas and tinctures. Although generally considered to be safe, do not confuse this herb with Chinese skullcap (*S. baicalensis*), which has totally different properties.

Slippery Elm

Ulmus fulva
Also known as sweet elm; moose elm; Indian elm

Before Dutch elm disease wiped out many of North America's mature trees, people tried using slippery elm's sweet-tasting inner bark to relieve many ailments—from diarrhea and rheumatism to coughs and ulcers.

Today, herbalists use slippery elm to treat inflammations, such as those that come with bladder infections, diarrhea, peptic ulcers, coughs, colitis, and acid stomach. You can apply homemade paste or gel to wounds or inflamed skin. You can also use the gel to restore vaginal lubrication during menopause. Herbalists say that it's the mucilage in slippery elm bark that helps with inflammation.

The inner bark of slippery elm is made into beverages and healing poultices. This herb is generally considered safe.

Valerian

Valeriana officinalis
Also known as all heal; moon root; great wild valerian

This showy plant with feathery pink blooms possesses such awful-smelling roots that the Greek physician Dioscorides nicknamed it "phu." But smelly or not, valerian has been used as a tranquilizer and anti-insomnia remedy for more than 1,000 years.

Valerian root reduces the time it takes to doze, lessens middle-of-the-night awakenings, and ensures groggy-free morning wake-ups. It also relaxes tense nerves and muscles, making it a natural choice for mood swings and menstrual cramps. Its compounds attach to the same brain receptors as tranquilizers like diazepam (Valium), but with milder effects and without the risk of addiction or dependence. Valerian also contains alkaloids that help lower blood pressure.

Take valerian root in teas, tinctures, tablets, or capsules. Do not take valerian with other sleep-enhancing or mood-controlling medications, such as Valium or amitriptyline (Elavil), since it can increase the effects of those drugs. Also, stop using it if you find yourself feeling stimulated, rather than calmed, by it. In some people, it may cause heart palpitations or nervousness.

WOMAN TO WOMAN
Battling Bouts of Insomnia

As an implementation consultant for a software company, Cheryl Carlile, 45, of St. Louis, Missouri, traveled nonstop. In just one week, she might travel from St. Louis to the East Coast, then to the West Coast, and then back to the Midwest. All this travel and time-zone hopping left her with sleeping problems, which sometimes turned into severe insomnia. Then she found someone who could help her. This is her story.

I traveled extensively for years, installing computer systems in hospitals, which is a very high stress environment. Between all the travel and the stress, I pretty much destroyed my natural sleeping patterns. Often I would lie there at night for hours, staring at the ceiling of a strange hotel room in a strange city.

At first, years and years ago, I got angry and frustrated, but the insomnia happened so often and for so long that I got used to it. I came to think of it as a normal condition. I could no longer recognize clues as to when I was tired and when I was awake.

Most people tend to wake up and go to sleep at the same times each day. They feel tired at bedtime, and they naturally wake up in the morning. I couldn't do either. I could be awake for two days and not feel tired. Then, once I finally did get to sleep, I wouldn't wake up unless someone roused me.

In hotel rooms, I would place a wake-up call *and* set an alarm, and sometimes still sleep right through both. Then I'd drift off during meetings. I wouldn't be noticeably sleeping, but my brain would shut down, and I wouldn't always be sure of what I was hearing.

Insomnia is this insidious thing. It creeps up on you, and you don't realize the effect it is having on your life until you get better. I didn't know how tired I was. I just functioned.

In looking for a remedy, I instinctively turned to herbs. My mother has always taken a very natural approach to health, so I am inclined to look into natural means as well. I met a trained, qualified herbalist, and she recommended some herbal solutions.

I now take valerian in conjunction with skullcap and passionflower. I take the herbs about an hour before I want to go to sleep because it takes a while for them to work. I can feel the valerian relax my muscles, and I start to get calm. The skullcap soothes my nerves, and the passionflower makes everything else work better for me. When I travel, I take all three herbs in pill or capsule form. If I am at home, I make a tea with everything but the valerian. I can't deal with valerian tea; it smells terrible. The next morning, I have absolutely no groggy feeling. I wake up and am refreshed, calm, and ready to go.

I'm really satisfied with the herbs I've been using. In fact, I don't think I could function without them.

Yarrow

Achillea millefolium
Also known as nosebleed; millefoil

Yarrow's Latin name comes from the ancient Greek hero Achilles. Its folk name, "nosebleed," refers to its ability to stop bleeding.

Yarrow, with its delicate white flowers and feathery green leaves, contains more than 120 compounds. It is used to reduce fevers, stop inflammation, control heavy menstrual flow, cool hot flashes, heal bladder infections, and relieve colds, flu, coughs, and sore throats. It's also used as a wash or a poultice to stop bleeding and heal wounds and in hot herbal baths to lessen menstrual cramps.

Take yarrow internally as a hot or cold tea, a tincture, or in capsules. In rare instances, handling its flowers can cause a skin rash.

Yellow Dock

Rumex crispus
Also known as curly dock; narrow-leaved dock

Depending on your point of view, yellow dock is vilified as a stubborn, unruly common weed or credited as a tonic for the bowels, liver, and skin. This long, golden-hued taproot first sprouted in Europe. It was brought to America by colonists.

Herbalists believe prolonged use of yellow dock lessens the effect of chronic skin problems such as acne, eczema, psoriasis, and rashes. The minerals in this herb also give a boost to women who feel tired all the time and offer relief as a gentle laxative. Yellow dock contains thiamin, iron, and vitamin C, plus compounds that stimulate bile production and nudge a sluggish liver, according to herb practitioners.

Yellow dock is best taken as a tea or tincture before meals, if you want to absorb its nutrients, and at bedtime for overnight constipation relief. It's also available in capsules. Yellow dock contains substances that may cause kidney stones, so consult a physician first before using it if you have a history of kidney stones.

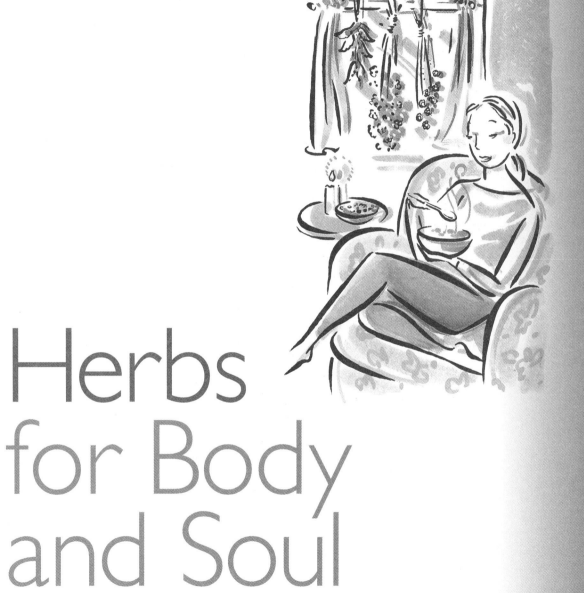

PART THREE

Herbs for Body and Soul

The Serenity Herbs

Take five minutes and say a prayer for yourself."

That's the advice of herbalist Kathleen Gould when she teaches her students about soothing teas. As masters of the Japanese tea ceremony have known for centuries, making tea involves much more than knowing how many teaspoons to use and how long to let the leaves steep. The making and drinking of an herbal tea should be a relaxing ritual.

"I always try to get my students to do some kind of ceremony," says Gould, a professional member of the American Herbalists Guild and director of the Herb Corner, an herbal teaching school in Indialantic, Florida.

Using herbs to relax and get rid of stress should be more than just taking medicine. It should be part of a rite that celebrates you. "If you are under chronic stress, you never get a break. Now do something for yourself. It is okay to do something for you," Gould says.

Many herbs contain substances that help bring on tranquillity and dissipate tension, and they have long been used to soothe away the stresses and strains that women undergo in their daily lives. But chemicals and compounds aren't the whole story. The process, the way you use herbs to calm, soothe, and relax, plays a major role in how they work.

Whether you're boiling water for tea, drawing a bath, or massaging your feet with herbal oil, there is something so soothing and peaceful in the act that it can be pure magic. "When you slow down enough to do this for yourself, you'll automatically start feeling a lot better," says Gail Ulrich, an herbalist, director of the Blazing Star Herbal School in Shelburne Falls, Massachusetts, and author of *Herbs to Boost Immunity*.

Women, in particular, need to take advantage of the refuge from daily life that an herbal bath or a soothing tea provides. "Women want to take care of everyone else. If we are stressed and nervous, we seem to deny ourselves first. Enjoying a bath, sipping a tea—these are ways of caring for ourselves as well as everyone else," Ulrich says.

Which herbs offer solace from a hectic world? Following are some well-known plants that are recommended by herbalists to help you calm down and relax.

Chamomile. In the nineteenth century, chamomile was used to treat the "nervousness" that sometimes accompanied a menstrual cycle. It's usually taken as a tea.

Lavender. The volatile oil in lavender, which contains more than 100 chemical compounds, calms the nervous system. It can be taken in a tea or tincture or used externally in baths and massage oils.

Lemon balm. Lemon balm calms tension, raises spirits, and relieves depression, insomnia, nervousness, and tension headaches. It's also known to pacify an upset stomach caused by stress. Lemon balm is usually used in tea or baths.

Oatstraw. This is a popular choice to allay tension headaches, insomnia, and nervous exhaustion. Oatstraw is mainly used as a tea and tincture.

Passionflower. This herb contains chemicals shown in laboratory studies to have sedating effects. It's often used to help bring on sleep and to ease the stress of premenstrual syndrome. Take it as a tea or tincture.

Skullcap. Thought to nourish the nervous system, this herb helps in times of stress. It also aids tension headaches, anxiety, depression, and exhaustion. It is used as a tea or tincture.

To use these serenity herbs correctly, create an accompanying serene atmosphere. All the lemon balm in the world won't calm you down if you are trying to feed the kids, open the mail, and do the

WOMAN TO WOMAN
She Brings Peace to Her Life

Linda Patterson, 34, of Winchendon, Massachusetts, leads a busy life. She's a professional herbalist who runs her own private practice, teaches at local schools, and runs conferences. She also devotes a great deal of her energy to volunteer work in her community. By the end of a hectic day, she's ready to relax, and she has her own special way of doing it.

My life is busy. Whose isn't? But it's also rich, full, and rewarding.

I do a lot of service work in the area where I live, and I spend a great deal of time working with the elderly. That's very satisfying, but it can also be pretty overwhelming and stressful. Older people are in great need sometimes, and there's only so much one person can do. I do what I can, but it never seems like enough. Then, like everyone else, I have bills to pay. Volunteer work doesn't exactly take care of them, so I also have to put as much time as I can into my profession. Juggling those two aspects of my life can really wear me down.

After a rough day, I love to relax by making tea. The sense of self-nurturing that comes with the act of making tea leaves me feeling at peace, and of course, sipping the hot tea afterward is probably the best relaxation I can think of.

When I get home, I head straight for the kitchen and start to boil water. Then I mix a tea of lemon balm and chamomile. Sometimes I throw in some dried rosemary. While it steeps, usually for about 10 minutes, I feed the dog or get a few things done, but mainly, I just enjoy the time.

Then it's time to set the scene. I put on some peaceful music, maybe George Winston or David Lanz. I gather what I need to do some creative writing—some paper, something to write with. I pour my tea. Then I curl up on my couch with my cup and sip. Its soothing heat helps me to write, and my writing helps me to relax. Within minutes, I can feel calmness come over me. Warming from the inside feels good. I just relax. The physical tension goes, then the mental tension goes. It is a great way to end the day.

dishes—all while the phone rings incessantly and the evening news blares from the TV.

Here's how to set the mood.

- Take your time. Whatever you are doing, don't rush it. Make sure you give yourself and the herb royal treatment. Celebrate each step of the process, even if it is something as simple as boiling the water, letting the herb steep, and straining the tea.
- Turn off the TV. Unplug the phone. Get rid of distractions.
- Light some candles. Play some soft music. Establish a relaxing ambience.
- Practice deep, slow breathing. That will help you relax and enjoy your herbal remedies.

Recipes for Relaxation

While tinctures, capsules, and teas of each individual serenity herb will help, there are many ways to mix and match them to create a wonderful soothing blend. Herbalists have devised many interesting and even fun ways to enjoy these calming herbs. Here's how you can use them, too.

Brew a calming cup. Sip a cup of this tea when you need to relax and wind down, says Jennifer Reid, N.D., a naturopathic physician in Gresham, Oregon. It combines several of the soothing serenity herbs. Mix 3 ounces of dried lemon balm, 1½ ounces of dried oatstraw, 1½ ounces of dried chamomile, ½ ounce of dried St. John's wort, ½ ounce of dried skullcap, and ½ ounce of dried passionflower. This recipe makes about 60 cups of tea. Boil 4 to 6 cups of water in a pot. After the water boils, add a tablespoon of the herb mixture for every 2 cups of water. Take the pot off the heat source and place a lid on it. Let it steep for 10 minutes. Then strain out the herbs and enjoy.

Steep your feet. If you put a lot of stress on

yourself, and especially your feet, take the pressure off both by making yourself an herbal footbath. Gould teaches herbal footbaths in her classes and says it is always a student favorite. "Footbaths work on so many levels. The scent, the colors, the heat," she says.

Good herbs for a relaxing footbath are dried roses (the leaves and petals), dried chamomile, and dried lavender. Boil one to two gallons of water in a pot. Add two cups of the herb mixture for each gallon of water. Cover it and let it cool. When it reaches a comfortable temperature—usually as hot as you can stand it—pour it into a small tub big enough for your feet.

Don't worry about straining the water; the pretty colors floating around your ankles add to the relaxing experience.

Soak in your tea. If it makes a good relaxing tea, it also makes a good relaxing bath. Leslie J. Peterson, N.D., a naturopathic physician in Orem, Utah, makes a relaxing tea of lemon balm, passionflower, and chamomile. Combine one-half ounce each of the three dried herbs. Use one teaspoon of the mixture for each cup of tea. Try the same combination of herbs in the tub for a soothing herbal bath blend. Make a gallon or so of the tea and pour it into your bath, she says. Then soak your cares of the day away.

Relax in a sea of salts. Toss in some homemade bath salts during your next long, hot bath, advises Gould. Take a cup of sea salts, which you can buy at a health food store, and place them in a glass jar. Add 10 drops of lavender essential oil and 10 drops of chamomile essential oil. Grab about one-half cup of the bath salts and add them to your bathwater.

"I enjoy using bath salts because they are calming and healing," Gould says.

One note of caution: Some essential oils, including those mentioned in this chapter, may cause skin irritation or an allergic reaction in certain individuals. People with sensitive skin should try a patch test before using essential oils.

Luxuriate in serenity bath oil. Ulrich created a "serenity bath oil" recipe that she says helps melt away stress and tension. Pour two ounces of almond or grapeseed oil into a jar or bottle. Add 10 drops of lavender essential oil, 10 drops of orange essential oil, and 2 to 3 drops of cedarwood essential oil. Shake well. Add one to two teaspoons of the bath oil into a full tub of water.

Mix an herbal cocktail. The herb damiana has a reputation as an aphrodisiac, but it also has the ability to quell anxiety, Gould says. To sit back and really relax with damiana, stir yourself up a sweet damiana elixir. Take a jar or bottle and fill it up halfway with dried damiana herb. Fill the rest of the bottle up with an alcoholic beverage of your choice, such as apricot brandy, peach schnapps, or banana liqueur to make the elixir tasty. Shake it a couple of times a day for two weeks. Leave it on your counter, out of direct sunlight, during this period, so you'll remember to shake it. Then strain the herb out of the liquid. Add a little bit of honey to sweeten the drink and mix it well. Finally, pour some of the elixir into a small cordial glass and sip. (Store the remainder away from direct sunlight and excessive heat.) "It is very calming to the central nervous system, and it is a great way to relax," Gould says.

Enjoy herbal popsicles. Remember taking your sweet time savoring a fruity popsicle as a kid? Why not use an herbal popsicle as a fun way to unwind at the end of the day. Instead of

THE HERBAL KITCHEN
Insomnia Tea

At one time or another, just about everyone has trouble getting to sleep, so every good herbalist has an insomnia tea recipe up her sleeve, says Shez Ward, an herbalist in Norfolk, England, and a member of the Royal Horticultural Society.

The following tea recipe, crafted by Ward, combines valerian, which is often recommended for insomnia, with skullcap and passionflower, which are used to relax and soothe.

Brew this tea about two hours before you go to bed. It takes about an hour to make, and you should start to feel sleepy within an hour after drinking it. One warning: Valerian has a bad odor and doesn't taste too pleasant, either. But it works.

- 1 cup water
- 3 teaspoons dried powdered valerian
- 1 teaspoon dried skullcap
- 2 teaspoons dried passionflower

Boil the water. Pour it into a cup containing the valerian, skullcap, and passionflower. Cover it and steep it for one hour. Strain the tea and add honey to taste. If you can't handle valerian in tea, take it in capsule form and make the tea without it, using two teaspoons of passionflower and three teaspoons of skullcap.

boiling water, boil apple juice, Gould says. Add one to two teaspoons of dried chamomile or dried lemon balm per cup of juice. Cover and let the herbs steep for 20 minutes. Strain the herbs from the juice. Pour the juice into an ice cube tray. Cover the tray with plastic wrap and place toothpicks in each cube. Place the ice cube tray in the freezer.

Knead away tension. Nothing takes away stress and puts you in a calmer mood better than a massage. Combine massage with some serenity herbs, and you double the relaxation. Let someone give you a massage, or treat yourself to a relaxing foot or hand massage with herb-infused oils.

To create a relaxing massage oil, choose one or a mix of the following herbs: dried roses, dried lavender, dried chamomile, and dried comfrey. Place two ounces of the mixture in a wide-mouth jar. Pour about one pint of almond, apricot, or grapeseed oil over the herbs so that there is at least two inches of oil above the herbs, says herbalist Rosemary Gladstar, director of the Sage Mountain Herbal Education Center in East Barre, Vermont, and author of *Herbal Healing for Women*. You may wish to add a drop or two of pure essential oil to scent the mixture. Let the jar sit in a warm place and shake it every day for two weeks. Using a kitchen strainer or a cheesecloth, strain the oil.

This supply will be enough for quite a few full-body massages, since you need to use only a small amount. Any remaining oil can be stored in your refrigerator for several months.

Spray worries away with lavender. Combine the soothing effects of lavender flowers with lavender essential oil in a floral spray. Mix ½ pint of distilled water with 1½ pints of white wine. Add in three-quarters teaspoon of lavender essential oil, and one tablespoon of dried lavender flowers. Let the mixture steep in a sunny window for three days, then put it in a cooler place for four days, Ulrich says. Strain out the dried herb and pour the mix into a spray bottle.

Spray your body or a room when you need a moment of relaxation, or add a cupful or two to bathwater. Store the solution in a cool spot away from light, such as in a cupboard.

Pack it in your purse. "You can't be living your life 90 miles an hour all day and then expect to take a teaspoon of something at night and be all better," Gould points out. Keep a bottle of a relaxing herbal tincture with a dropper in your purse. Try a combination of chamomile and passionflower, for example. Every few hours, take a few dropperfuls of the tincture in water or juice. "Slowly let your body relax throughout the day," she says.

The Energizing Herbs

All of us know at least one really perky person. She's the one who gets up earlier than we do, exercises every day, gets "most valuable employee" awards at work, cooks a gourmet meal for her husband and three kids every night, coaches the girls' soccer team, canvasses for an environmentalist group, takes ballroom dancing lessons, is never out of breath, never looks tired, and always has a smile on her face. She reminds you of that whack-a-mole game you see in arcades: You can't keep her down!

She was obviously born that way. The rest of us may not have been so lucky. We know the meaning of fatigue. Our kids and grandkids frazzle us. The office grind or housekeeping battles can turn us into 5:00 P.M. zombies. We hang on by our fingernails, yearning for the weekends, as if our dream of sleeping late on Saturday morning will ever really come true. We feel doomed to low energy.

But we're not.

There's something we can do.

If you should ever find yourself doing lunch with a group of herbalists, something will strike you immediately: You're surrounded by perky people. Despite busy, on-the-go lives— moving from one conference to the next, crossing time zones, delivering lectures, keeping up with new findings, creating new formulas—herbalists manage to remain energized and enthusiastic.

And here's the interesting part: Most of them weren't born that way!

Obviously, they're on to something. But it's not wizardry. It's basic knowledge of the human body, plus some common sense, and—you guessed it—a few herbs.

Here's what we know: There are three bad guys in the body that rob us of our energy: toxins, infections, and hormonal imbalances. The liver should take care of toxins; the immune system should stamp out infections; and the endocrine system should keep our hormones in balance. And they all do—so long as we keep them healthy and well-cared-for.

How do we do that? To begin with, by making sound dietary and lifestyle choices, such as getting enough sleep, exercising regularly, and eating plenty of fresh fruits, vegetables, and whole-grain products.

Once these fundamental healthy behaviors are

WOMAN TO WOMAN

A Busy Mother Recharges Her Life

Brenda Van Natta, a shiatsu practitioner, herbalist, and mother of two from Easton, Pennsylvania, went through a period in her life when her immune system seemed to declare a work slowdown. Constant illness and infection were draining her vigor away. But she didn't give up. Instead, she made a decision that turned her life around. Here is her story.

There came a time in my life when I found I could no longer summon up the energy I needed to cope from day to day. To make matters worse, I was sick all the time. You name it, I got it: colds, strep throat, bladder infections, even an ovarian cyst. And I couldn't make it through a winter without coming down with bronchitis.

I tried decongestants, cold formulas, and antibiotics, but they left me feeling dizzy and throbbing with headaches. After a while, they seemed to stop working altogether. I thought I would simply have to accept all that sickness as a way of life.

If it weren't for my little boy, Jimmy, I might have gone on that way indefinitely. Like me, he had been getting sick all the time, and he was on medication. But when *his* prescriptions also stopped working, I decided that enough was enough. I couldn't watch my little boy go through that. I turned to herbs.

I read several books about herbs, which recommended that Jimmy and I take echinacea for colds. It helped immediately. I could hardly believe it. In fact, I felt so inspired that I began taking classes with herbalist David Winston.

Looking back, I'd have to say that herbs saved my life. As for Jimmy, he's now active in soccer and scouts.

Of course, I've made other changes in my life as well. I've learned healthier ways to eat and drink. I used to order extra cheese on my pizza and drink up to five cups of coffee a day. Now, I've eliminated dairy products and coffee from my diet. Refined sugar, too. I now drink green tea with honey and lemon.

With herbs, I've gone from being sick and tired to functioning at my best. Now, I have all the pep I need for my son, Jimmy, and my daughter, Niki.

in place, herbal healers say you can use herbs to put more spring in your step and keep your energy high all day. They can help to fortify your liver, bolster your immune system, and keep your hormones in balance.

"We encourage women to take a holistic approach to improving their health," says Mindy Green, a founding and professional member of the American Herbalists Guild, director of educational services for the Herb Research Foundation in Boulder, Colorado, and coauthor of *Aromatherapy: A Complete Guide to the Healing Art.* "Herbal remedies restore energy best when women discontinue abusive behaviors like drinking coffee and smoking cigarettes."

Here are some ways that herbalists keep themselves going strong.

Swap coffee for green tea. If you need a morning wake-up, try green tea. It contains caffeine, but it also has beneficial compounds you won't find in coffee.

"Green tea gives you energy and added benefits, such as antioxidants, that round up free radicals in your cells," says Green, a regular green tea drinker. "I advise steeping the green tea for no more than three minutes, or it will taste bitter. Adding a bit of honey to sweeten it is fine."

If you're in a hurry, keep a supply of organic green tea bags on hand. If you want to make it yourself, infuse one teaspoon of organic dried green tea leaves into a cup of boiling water for a few minutes, then strain out the leaves and sip.

Bounce back from sleepless nights. If you find yourself dragging through your morning because you tossed and turned all of the previous night, Green suggests trying a traditional Chinese medicine called schisandra. This herb has been used for centuries for insomnia and physical exhaustion. You can find it in health food stores or order it through the mail.

For tea drinkers, use one teaspoon of crushed powder per cup of boiling water. Steep the powder for 10 to 20 minutes, then strain and sip. Drink up to three cups a day to revive your energy.

If you'd rather take schisandra in capsules, the recommended daily amount is 1,500 to 6,000 milligrams split in two doses.

Restore energy with dandelion. That common nuisance of a weed blooming in the cracks of your sidewalk can be a real pal in helping you get the poisons out of your system. "The dandelion root is considered one of the supreme herbs for the liver," says herbalist Rosemary Gladstar, director of the Sage Mountain Education Center in East Barre, Vermont, and author of *Herbal Healing for Women.*

Loaded with vitamins and minerals, both its root and leaves can help your liver to do a better job of ridding toxins from your body.

Gladstar enjoys sipping dandelion tea or eating a salad abundant with fresh dandelion leaves on a daily basis.

Send fatigue fleeing with an uplifting tea. When your on-the-go lifestyle finds you skipping meals or ordering too many dinners at the drive-up window, your body craves recharging. Try reducing or eliminating feelings of fatigue with this tea prepared by Gladstar.

Collect two parts of raspberry leaf, two parts of nettle leaf, four parts of peppermint, one part of alfalfa, and one-quarter part of grated gingerroot. Scoop four to six tablespoons of this herbal blend into a quart of cold water in a saucepan.

Bring the tea to a simmer over low heat with the pan covered. Remove the pan from the stove, and allow the tea to sit for 20 minutes. Strain out the herbs, and drink up to four cups a day.

Gain energy with ginseng. If you're seeking an herb that can go the distance in helping your body overcome stress and fatigue, then consider Siberian ginseng. This herb seems to especially rejuvenate women going through menopause by stepping in as a hormonal leveler and mood enhancer, says Gladstar.

Although there are many ways to take ginseng, Gladstar enjoys making a tonic using fresh Siberian ginseng root. Cut a four-inch ginseng root into slices. Tuck the slices in a small glass jar with four cups of water and seal it with a lid. Place the jar in a large pot with enough water to cover about three-fourths of the jar. Cover the pot with a lid; simmer slowly for about six hours. Add water if the level gets below one-half. This method provides you with a concentrated ginseng tonic that will help end your energy drain. You need only take it once or twice a month.

For best results, drink a cup of this ginseng tonic at night with a light meal of grains and steamed vegetables. If needed, you can drink another cup in the morning, says Gladstar.

Dine on stimulating soup. When a cold or flu zaps you of your energy and taxes your immune system, consider this herbal soup created by Jennifer Reid, N.D., a naturopathic physician in Gresham, Oregon.

In a vegetable broth base, combine two handfuls of fresh parsley, one large shiitake mushroom (sliced), three slices of fresh ginger, three garlic cloves, and one-quarter teaspoon of cayenne pepper. You can also add sliced carrots or other favorite soup vegetables. Simmer in a covered pot for 10 minutes. Have up to three cups a day to fend off energy-draining colds and flu.

Cayenne can irritate your gastrointestinal

WOMEN ASK WHY

Since I'm convinced that using herbs is the best way to safeguard my health, should I give up taking vitamin and mineral supplements?

Herbs work in concert with vitamins and minerals. They don't replace them. Used together, they correct deficiencies and imbalances in the basic chemistry of your body. Because of that, they can be very powerful in dealing with women's health issues.

Women entering menopause, for instance, can achieve tremendous health benefits from taking calcium and magnesium citrate to help prevent and treat osteoporosis. At the same time, black cohosh works effectively to relieve many menopausal symptoms, including hot flashes and interrupted sleep.

For symptoms of PMS, vitamin B_6 can help regulate hormone pathways and aid the liver in clearing estrogen out of the body. I also believe that vitex (also known as chasteberry) is one of the most effective herbs for balancing female hormones.

The only way to decide which herbs and supplements you should be taking is by determining your individual needs. What is your age and medical condition? What is your diet like? Is there anything in your family history that might be important to consider? It's always a good idea to consult with a medical expert who can provide guidelines for combining herbs with vitamins and minerals. When you do, bring in the bottles of vitamins and minerals you're already taking.

Even in combination with vitamin supplements, herbs don't produce immediate results. These natural medicines take time, sometimes weeks, even months, to work effectively on your body's system. But the benefits can last a lifetime.

Expert consulted
Angela Stengler, N.D.
Naturopathic physician
Coauthor of Menopause Relief: Nature's
    Top Herbal Medicines and More
Oceanside, California

tract if you take it on an empty stomach.

This nutrient-rich and calorie-low soup is hot and spicy, says Dr. Reid. The garlic and mushrooms fight bacterial and viral invaders; ginger and cayenne pepper aid digestion; and parsley is high in iron and vitamin C.

Keep pace with a stamina formula. If you enjoy working out at the gym; taking long, brisk walks; or spending hours in the garden, you may want to try the following stamina formula for active women and men, created by herbalist Kathi Keville, director of the American Herb Association and author of *Herbs for Health and Healing*.

Combine one teaspoon of Siberian ginseng root tincture with one-half teaspoon each of tinctures of schisandra berries, ginseng root (American or Korean), saw palmetto berries, and licorice root. Take half a dropperful twice a day, or as needed to boost your stamina.

Ginseng and schisandra seem to help improve endurance, muscle strength, cardiovascular fitness, and mental clarity. Licorice appears to increase energy storage in your muscles, while saw palmetto may aid in building muscles.

Smart Healing with Herbs

Columbus discovered America by accident. He wasn't after real estate. He was after herbs.

Queen Isabella . . . trade route to India . . . herbs and spices. . . . Every American school-child knows the story. But exactly what made these herbs so desirable that men would risk their lives plying the briny deeps to get them? The same thing that makes modern medicines so valuable: their curative powers.

Today, we can get even the rarest herbs through the mail or at the health food store down the street. But availability isn't enough. Knowing how to use them is just as important.

If you are socked with a nagging headache but are reluctant to keep reaching for the bottle of ibuprofen, what else can you take? If you feel a cold coming on but you dread the drowsiness delivered from the over-the-counter capsule, is there a better alternative? If you need an energy boost but know that coffee isn't a healthy choice, what is healthier and works as well?

Try taming that throbbing head with white willow. Calm the cold with echinacea. Fend off fatigue with a whiff of peppermint. The knowledge of how to use herbs is an ancient wisdom that women are now beginning to rediscover.

"Women have found that using herbs frees them from many of the side effects they were experiencing with their prescription medications," says Jennifer Reid, N.D., a naturopathic physician in Gresham, Oregon. "Herbs can be powerful yet gentle to the body if used in the proper way."

All of this brings up an interesting question. When you think about ginger and garlic, are they foods or are they medicines? "The answer is that it really depends on how they are delivered, how much you're taking, and how often. Everything is dosage," answers Mindy Green, a founding and professional member of the American Herbalists Guild, director of educational services for the Herb Research Foundation in Boulder, Colorado, and coauthor of *Aromatherapy: A Complete Guide to the Healing Art*.

When herbs are used as a remedy, one basic rule always applies: Although usually quite safe, they must still be treated with the same caution that is applied to prescription and over-the-counter medications. Beyond that, care must be taken in choosing the right herb in the right form and in the right dose. For instance, ginkgo makes a great-tasting tea, but if you're looking to sharpen your memory, a standardized extract capsule is the best medicinal choice, says Green.

"At times, herbs can be used instead of a drug that has harmful side effects," says Dr. Reid. Sometimes herbs can complement prescription medication. Whichever way they are used, it's best if the choice of herb or herbs is formulated to fit the specific needs of the individual.

Check with your doctor before taking herbs in place of your prescription medications, especially those for chronic conditions such as diabetes or high blood pressure. Also, get your physician's stamp of approval before you add herbs to your medications in the hope of achieving better results. If you're taking a digitalis-type medication for your heart condition, for example, you could develop serious problems by adding hawthorn.

Rarely do women develop side effects from taking herbs. But if you suddenly develop skin rashes, forehead-tapping headaches, mild diarrhea, or nausea lasting longer than two days, your body might be telling you that it doesn't want these substances. Work with a health practitioner qualified in the use of herbal remedies to determine if these symptoms mean you need to reduce the amount of herb, change the specific formula, or switch to a different formula altogether.

Two special cautions: Stop using herbs as soon as you know you are pregnant. And everyone needs to practice extra caution when using essential oils—extracts distilled from the roots, resins, bark, wood, fruit, leaves, and flowers of plants. Potent and complex, essential oils should *never* be swallowed because ingesting even a few drops can be toxic. They are best used externally in diluted forms. The few exceptions are noted in the chart at the end of this book.

The herbal remedies offered by qualified professionals for the health conditions that follow are readily available at health food stores, from mail-order catalogs, and in some cases, even at your local supermarket or drugstore. They were selected because they are easy to use or simple to make. More important, top herbalists and alternative medicine experts regard them as safe with little, if any, side effects.

Acne

You thought you'd left acne behind when you graduated from high school, but the truth is, acne isn't just kids' stuff. Skin problems can continue or make a comeback in your thirties, forties, and fifties. Why? Too much sebum, an oily substance secreted by glands in your skin. Sebum collects dirt and bacteria, clogging pores. Hormonal fluctuations (right before your menstrual period or as you approach menopause), stress, fatty diets, and even the harsh ingredients in some cosmetics can shift your sebum production into high gear.

The result? A variety of blemish types. If a tiny hair follicle becomes plugged, you get a whitehead. When this plug rises to the skin's surface and meets the air, it darkens and becomes a blackhead. Should the blockage become inflamed, infected, or ruptured, you get the frustrating, sometimes painful eruptions known as cystic acne.

Herbalists recommend attacking acne in two ways. First, control it from the inside out with herbs that may help your body eliminate waste material more effectively and bring your hormones to normal levels when you're having your period or during menopause. Second, use gentle but effective herbal cleansers and moisturizers. Try these techniques recommended by herbal experts.

For cleansing, take root. Burdock root has a long tradition of use for skin problems. Herbalists believe it works by helping the liver eliminate waste more effectively. Take one capsule of dried burdock or 30 drops of burdock root tincture with meals three times a day. Or make a batch of strong burdock tea. Use one teaspoon of dried, chopped burdock root per cup of boiling water. Steep at least 10 to 20 minutes, then strain and sip. Steeping overnight makes an even stronger brew. Have a cup or two daily to fight acne.

Increase bile flow with dandelion. A common backyard "weed," dandelion actually has a long-held reputation as a cleansing herb. It contains bitter compounds that can increase bile flow and stimulate the liver. The benefit? Your body eliminates waste more efficiently, which leads to clearer skin. Some herbalists suggest you take a teaspoon of dandelion tincture daily, diluted in eight ounces of water. Sip part in the morning, part later in the day, and the rest in the evening.

Cleanse with oatmeal. Make a daily habit of removing dirt and excess oil from your face—gently. Wash your face with an unscented oatmeal soap. Or prepare a simple oatmeal scrub by grinding old-fashioned or instant rolled oats in a food processor, clean coffee grinder, or a blender. Mix two teaspoons of the oats with about one tablespoon of water to form a paste. Gently wash your face with the mixture, then rinse with warm or lukewarm water. In either form, oatmeal removes dirt and oil without stripping all the natural oils from your skin.

Fight bacteria with lavender essential oil. Restore a clear complexion by placing one or two drops of pure essential oil of lavender directly on your blemish as needed. Unlike most essential oils, lavender can be applied "neat," meaning it can be used directly on the skin in small amounts, without having to be diluted in a carrier oil. Lavender oil is great for a variety of skin conditions because it attacks bacteria and eases pain and swelling.

Moisturize to prevent breakouts. A light moisturizer actually helps acne-prone skin. Mix a drop or two of lavender essential oil into an ounce of light oil such as jojoba or sunflower, and apply at night. Why add oil to skin that's already breaking out? Herbal beauty experts say moisturized skin is less likely to overproduce oil and be at risk for acne.

ALOE
Good for: minor skin rashes, scrapes, cuts, and burns

Age Spots

Despite the name, age spots may have more to do with overexposure to the sun than the accumulation of birthdays. These dark brown blotches—also called liver spots—that appear on a woman's skin are the result of years of sun exposure.

When the prime targets—the face, neck, chest, forearms, and hands—are bombarded by the sun's ultraviolet light day after day, year after year, the skin responds by producing melanin, a naturally dark pigment. At first, age spots usually look just like freckles or small moles. Over time, though, they can darken, grow, and multiply, especially if you keep exposing them to the sun.

Dermatologists advise women to wear sunscreen and avoid the sun to reduce the occurrence of new age spots and the continued growth of existing spots. Herbal beauty experts suggest going two steps further: First, use herbal treatments that safely fade and peel away the upper layer of overpigmented, blotchy skin. Then, apply moisturizing formulas that promote the growth of new skin cells, which can make skin look fresher.

Peel sun damage away with elder-flowers. In combination, lemon juice and fresh or dried elderflowers will help bleach and remove age spots over time. Both contain alpha hydroxy acids that stimulate peeling of the skin's upper layer. Age spots fade and, over time, slough away as natural acids loosen old, dead cells and surface discoloration.

Combine one tablespoon of fresh or dried elderflowers and one teaspoon of lemon juice, and mix in a food processor or blender. Add just enough water to form a paste. Apply with your fingers to the age spots, being careful to avoid your eyes and lips. It may sting a bit. Leave the paste on for no more than five minutes, then rinse it off with lukewarm water. Apply three times per week. Expect to see age spots fade within three months.

Peel with parsley. You can also create an effective face peel using lemon juice, a little water, and chopped parsley in place of elderflowers. Follow the directions above for making and using this all-natural peel.

Allergies

If you've ever had a sneezing attack while vacuuming or grooming your cat, you may have blamed the stirred-up dust and fur. But allergists say the real culprit is your own immune system, which is overreacting to the dust and dander—and provoking all those a-a-a-choos.

Allergies are abnormal reactions to everyday substances like dust mites, pet dander, and mold spores. When your immune system misidentifies these harmless substances as dangerous invaders, your body goes overboard in releasing invasion-fighting chemicals including histamine. Histamine produces the symptoms of an allergic reaction: sniffles, skin inflammation, indigestion, and headache. In rare cases, usually involving food, drug, or insect allergies, it can even cause a life-threatening body-wide reaction, complete with breathing difficulties and a dangerous plunge in blood pressure.

Standard medical care for most allergies calls for decongestants, antihistamines, and, sometimes, allergy shots. The decongestants open clogged nasal passages. Antihistamines block the effect of histamine. And allergy shots slowly expose your body to substances it reacts to so that you gradually become desensitized.

Although effective, some of these medications can cause drowsiness, insomnia, and, in some people, raised blood pressure. Herbalists and alternative medical experts suggest using the following safe plant remedies instead. If you find that your symptoms of sneezing, wheezing, or coughing aren't reduced by these remedies or over-the-counter medicines you've tried, it might be time to visit your doctor.

Dry out watery eyes with eyebright. If allergies leave you with weepy, watery eyes, turn to eyebright. Herbalists say this herb naturally tones and strengthens the ocular membranes behind the eyes and can stop eye-watering. Take one to four milligrams of eyebright as a tincture three times a day, as needed.

Breathe easy with ginkgo. The ginkgo tree, often planted in Japanese temple gardens, has an ancient reputation for bolstering the kidneys, lungs, and digestive system and for restoring vitality. Used by some natural healers specifically for allergies, ginkgo contains compounds called ginkgolides that may counter spasms of the bronchial muscles when your immune system is exposed to an allergen like pollen or animal dander. As a result, you can breathe comfortably instead of wheezing. Take 20 to 30 drops of ginkgo tincture up to four times a day. You can dilute the dose in water, juice, or herbal tea.

Season with garlic. Garlic contains high concentrations of the compound quercetin, noted for reducing the severity of inflammatory reactions. If you have allergies, add generous amounts of garlic to your meals.

Altitude Sickness

"Breathtaking" may describe panoramic views from pristine mountaintops, but fast climbs, mountain drives, or even ski-lift rides can also take your breath away.

Altitude sickness is related directly to elevation. At sea level, oxygen molecules in your blood are dense and rich. But at 16,000 feet above sea level, your blood contains one-third less oxygen. When your body is deprived of adequate oxygen, your brain, heart, lungs, and nervous system are affected. Without proper precautions, you may develop dizziness, breathlessness, fatigue, headaches, nausea, and even vomiting. The higher and faster you climb, the worse the symptoms may become.

Fortunately, you can minimize, or even avoid, altitude sickness by working in harmony with Mother Nature's medicinal garden. Just as you prepare in advance for a mountain hike by packing the right gear and supplies, you can prepare your body by taking these herbal fortifiers a few days before your next sky-high adventure begins.

Stave off stress with Siberian ginseng. Walking, skiing, or simply vacationing in high-altitude terrain can be quite an adjustment, especially if you normally reside at low altitudes. Start preparing your body a few days before any cloud-climbing expedition by taking Siberian ginseng capsules. This herb, called an adaptogen by herbalists, will bolster your body's resistance to stress, especially environmental stress. Check the bottle's label for dosage information.

Sip a spicy garlic soup. Before that next mountain hike or ski trip to the big slopes, spoon up this herbal soup and forestall altitude-related discomfort. Simply combine generous amounts of fresh garlic, dill, fennel, tomatoes, onions, hot peppers, canned soybeans (they'll cook faster than dried), celery, carrots, and parsley in a few cups of water and simmer for 20 minutes or so. Garlic is the key, but all these ingredients work together to help keep your blood from thickening as you gain altitude.

Keep a clear head with ginkgo. Increase your chances for a trip free of headaches and dizziness by taking 120 milligrams of standardized ginkgo extract daily for several days beforehand. Studies have demonstrated that ginkgo leaves make blood vessels in the brain more flexible, allowing for better circulation. Ginkgo also thins the blood, helping reduce headaches and dizziness by supplying more oxygen to the brain.

Anemia

A woman with anemia may feel weary and weak. The simplest activities, such as folding laundry, making dinner, driving to the office, or just helping the kids with their homework, become energy-sapping.

What's going on? The answer may be in your blood. Anemia is the medical term for a reduction in red blood cell count. Red blood cells contain hemoglobin, a protein that transports oxygen to muscles, body tissues, and organs—where it fortifies and energizes. Without sufficient red blood cells, your body won't receive enough oxygen to function optimally, leaving you feeling tired, cold, lousy, and lifeless.

BASIL
Good for: diarrhea without any other symptoms and fever associated with colds and flu

While there are several types of anemia, the most common variety among women is iron-deficiency anemia. Inside red blood cells, iron atoms bind with oxygen. The cells then deliver the iron throughout the body. When your iron levels drop—because of menstruation, pregnancy, childbirth, crash diets, or perpetual weight-watching, for example—your body makes fewer or smaller red blood cells, with less hemoglobin. As a result, there's less oxygen—leaving you exhausted. (Iron-deficiency anemia is rare among women who have been through menopause. In fact, after menopause a woman may have to worry more about having too much iron.)

How do you know if you're anemic? A simple blood test is the best indicator.

Conventional doctors often prescribe iron supplements in the form of ferrous sulfate to treat iron-deficiency anemia. Some herbal experts, however, say these supplements may not be fully absorbed by the body and can cause constipation and stomach distress. If you take these supplements for prolonged periods, say some herbalists, they may spark the formation of free radicals, oxygen-stealing molecules that contribute to such diseases as colon cancer and heart disease.

Instead of iron supplements, bolster your diet with dark green leafy vegetables and foods that are naturally rich in iron such as roasted dark turkey meat or steamed clams. Then supplement those smart food choices with some of these herbal remedies.

Boost iron with yellow dock root. This bitter-tasting herb is believed by some herbalists to be the best herbal antidote for iron deficiency. Try commercially made yellow dock capsules, following label directions. Some women find that their iron levels return to normal within a few weeks to a month.

Brew an iron-rich tea. Fortify your body's iron supply by drinking two cups of this "iron tea" each day. Mix two teaspoons yellow dock root with one-half teaspoon each of nettle leaves, dandelion root, beet root, and licorice root. Boil this herbal blend in three cups of water. Then turn down the heat and simmer the mixture on the stove for 5 minutes. Turn off the heat and let it steep for another 20 minutes. Strain out the herbs before drinking the tea.

Munch a dandelion-dressed salad. Fresh dandelion leaves contain iron as well as magnesium, which assists your body in using iron more efficiently. Make a tasty salad dressing by cutting several handfuls of dandelion leaves (only use leaves from a pesticide-free yard). Rinse them free of dirt and toss into a blender. Add oil, vinegar, and herbs and spices of your choice. Blend until the mixture is pureed. Then pour over a salad loaded with kale, spinach, parsley, and other dark leafy greens.

Anxiety

If women were clairvoyant, we'd never feel anxious. After all, anxiety is the dread of the not-yet-known. It's that churning sensation in the pit of your stomach when the phone rings unexpectedly at 4:00 A.M., that mounting tension when the plumber mutters his third "Hmmmm" while examining your kitchen sink.

Lingering anxiety blocks concentration and ignites irritability and sleepless nights—as well as chip-and-dip feeding frenzies. Unchecked, anxiety can elevate your blood pressure and heart rate and make you more susceptible to serious conditions, such as heart disease.

If the anxiety you're feeling is so overwhelming that you are severely distressed, can't enjoy yourself, or can no longer handle the responsibilities of your day-to-day life, it's a good idea to check with a medical doctor or professional psychotherapist.

You can begin controlling mild or moderate anxiety, however, with calm breathing. When you're anxious, you may breathe shallowly or even hold your breath. By contrast, slow, deep breathing will calm your nervous system. So take a deep breath—then, rely on these herbal helpers to help you ditch the jitters.

Restore calm with valerian. Soothe an overly excited nervous system by taking one to two capsules (100 to 300 milligrams each) or 30 to 60 drops of valerian tincture three times a day. Doctors of alternative medicine routinely prescribe valerian in place of diazepam (Valium), alprazolam (Xanax), or other prescription drugs for mild and moderate cases of anxiety.

Rely on kava kava. To subdue feelings of fear and anger, try kava kava, a tropical plant that thrives in the humid South Pacific. Kava kava contains kavalactones, a group of resinous compounds that relax mind and body. Take one capsule (100 milligrams) or 30 drops of standardized kava root tincture three times a day during anxious times. Studies have shown that kava acts on the limbic system, the emotional control center of the brain, subduing feelings of fear and anger while enhancing feelings of pleasure.

Sniff out anxiety with angelica essential oil. If you're prone to feeling anxious, prevent those uneasy feelings from mushrooming into a panic attack by keeping a bottle of angelica essential oil handy. The essential oil extracted from this

WOMAN TO WOMAN
She Overcame Anxiety with Kava Kava

Eileen Roche, 46, a professor of nursing from Media, Pennsylvania, was diagnosed with an aggressive form of breast cancer in her early forties. Although she beat the disease and is now cancer-free, Eileen still experiences bouts of anxiety whenever she visits her oncologist, especially if he orders tests. To overcome her anxiety, Eileen started taking kava kava, which enables her to control her fears instead of them controlling her.

At a very young age, 41, I was diagnosed with inflammatory breast cancer. That particular form of the disease is extremely lethal and has a low survival rate. But I was lucky. I went through treatment, and the cancer went into remission. So far, I'm a breast cancer survivor.

Still, because the disease was so aggressive and I was so young, I'm anxious that it might come back. I routinely visit an oncologist for checkups, of course, but going there is nerve-racking. Even thinking about seeing my doctor, who's a sweet guy, gets me all worked up: I'm not able to sleep, my stomach gets tense, and I can feel the anxiety building.

The worst part is when he orders tests. I immediately start to get anxious about what the results are going to be. I think of all the potential problems over and over. I read the statistics, and I worry about my chances of getting cancer again. It's like a broken record. I just want it to stop.

Kava does that. It makes it stop.

I had already been reading about herbs, and I remembered having seen something about treating anxiety with kava. I decided to give it a try. The results were wonderful. Even with all of my anxiety surrounding doctor visits, it completely settled me. After taking kava, I felt calmer and could sleep. It also kept me from worrying about everything over and over again. And it didn't make me drowsy. It just took the edge off.

Now I start to take kava about a week before my oncologist visit—that's usually when all of the worry begins to seep in and build up—and I'm able to function normally. When the visit is done and all the related tests and questions are settled, I simply stop taking it.

Based on my experience, I highly recommend kava to others.

herb restores calm and composure. Put a drop of angelica oil on a hankie and sniff its healing aroma whenever you feel your anxiety escalating.

Arthritis

If you picture a hunched-over, knobby-jointed grandmother when you think of arthritis, take another look. The real picture is this: Arthritis pain knows no age limits. More than 100 types can affect women at all stages of life—from grandmothers to mothers to daughters.

Two of the most common forms, osteoarthritis and rheumatoid arthritis, don't usually bother women until their forties. Osteoarthritis, the wear-and-tear type, erodes the soft, spongy cartilage that cushions joints, leading to joint pain and stiffness. Rheumatoid arthritis, on the other hand, is an autoimmune disease that prompts the body's own immune system to turn on itself. It causes the membrane that lubricates each joint to swell. Other symptoms of rheumatoid arthritis include redness in the joints, fever, fatigue, and loss of appetite.

Having arthritis does not necessarily mean enduring a lifetime of pain. Eating healthfully and making other lifestyle changes can soften the symptoms. Certain herbs can also improve mobility and reduce pain and stiffness.

Rub down with lemon and sandalwood. An herbal rub made with essential oils can ease joint pain and inflammation. Make your own by starting with a small jar of petroleum jelly. Scoop out a tablespoon of the jelly. Then add 20 drops of essential oil of lemon and 20 drops of essential oil of sandalwood to the jar. Mix the oil well

WOMAN TO WOMAN
Herbal Answers for Her Arthritis

June Godfrey thought she had dodged a bullet. She was in her midseventies, and she had never had a hint of arthritis. Then it struck. The effect it had on her hands, hips, and knees was devastating. Her prescription medications helped a little, but not enough. Still, she didn't give up. She found another way to deal with her pain. This is her story.

Every year, Washington's rainy season seems to seep into my bones, and arthritis puts me in a foul temper. I was 77 when I first began to feel the inflammation in the joints of my hands. Because I had reached my seventies without any sign of the disease, I thought I wasn't going to have to go through it. Now look: I'm the subject of an arthritis profile in this book.

During the five or six years that I've had arthritis, my knees and hips have given me the most pain. I first went to my regular doctor for some relief. He prescribed pills that took the sharp edge off, but my quality of life still wasn't everything it could have been.

I had tremendous trouble going from a standing to a sitting position or vice versa, and not being able to sleep through the night stole the luster from my life. Life isn't as

into the petroleum jelly. Rub this mixture on sore joints four times a day.

Improve joint mobility with ginger. Ginger's anti-inflammatory qualities may help curb the pain, swelling, and morning stiffness often associated with rheumatoid arthritis. Slice a piece of fresh ginger. Put a few slivers into a tea ball. Place the tea ball in a cup, pour freshly boiled water over it, and steep for 10 minutes. Make sure the tea has cooled to a comfortable temperature before sipping.

Stimulate the liver and kidneys with two roots. Herbalists believe that arthritis may improve when the body eliminates wastes more effun when you're too sleepy and achy to visit with friends or do many of the things that you once did.

For most of my life, I hadn't used herbs for anything but cooking, but three years ago, my late husband had a stroke, and we consulted an herbalist who worked with my husband's conventional doctor to help him recover. During her visits to my husband, our herbalist, Gayle Eversole, began to treat my arthritis as well. She prescribed a handful of supplements to help relieve my swollen joints.

It's been sort of trial and error finding the right combination of herbs, vitamins, and minerals. But a few herbs markedly improved the way I felt: garlic, ginger, and valerian. The garlic and ginger are wonderful because they help reduce my achiness and swelling. But valerian is my favorite because its relaxing properties help me sleep through the night. Every day for the past three years, I've faithfully taken these herbs because they're a large part of the reason I can function again.

Now, I'm able to walk a half block to have dinner with my friends. It takes me 24 minutes to make that walk, but I do it because exercise helps keep the arthritis at bay and because I refuse to become addicted to a wheelchair. I'm also taking less than half as many pain pills. My doctor is amazed at how healthy I seem. Best of all, though, life is rich again, and I'm happier.

ficiently. To achieve this, they turn to burdock and dandelion, which encourage healthy liver and kidneys. Try this anti-arthritis tea: Boil one teaspoon of dried dandelion root and one teaspoon of dried burdock root in three cups of water for five minutes. Strain and sip throughout the day. If the taste is too bitter for your liking, add a bit of honey.

Suppress the pain with cayenne. Place a dash of cayenne pepper on the tip of your tongue, and it feels like a three-alarm fire is blazing inside your mouth. But apply this red pepper herb in cream form to an achy elbow, knee, or other arthritic joint, and it may make pain disappear. Cayenne contains two important ache-fighting chemicals: capsaicin and salicylates. Capsaicin relieves pain by unleashing endorphins, your body's homemade feel-good chemicals. Salicylates have aspirin-like properties. Apply capsaicin cream directly to painful arthritic joints four times daily. Always thoroughly wash your hands afterward to avoid getting the cream in your eyes.

Asthma

Some things set women up for trouble with asthma. Classic asthma-attack triggers include exposure to air pollutants, pet dander, pollen, or mold, or a bad cold, exercise, stress, crying, anger, or even hearty laughter. Hormone fluctuations during menstruation or pregnancy may also cause heightened asthma symptoms for some sensitive women.

No matter the cause of your asthma, the scenario inside your lungs is the same: During an attack, the tubes that allow oxygen to pass into your lungs tighten and swell. At the same time, these passages produce a lot of mucus, which further clogs airways. Breathing becomes difficult, and you may wheeze, cough, or feel tightness in your chest.

Asthma should never be ignored: It's important to see your doctor for a treatment plan. She's likely to prescribe drugs that will quickly relax constricted breathing passages and reduce inflammation. You should never stop taking your asthma medication without your doctor's approval. That said, you may be able to reduce your dependence on these medications and breathe easier with the following herbal treatments.

Go for ginkgo. For centuries, Asian healers have relied on extracts of ginkgo leaves to safely treat asthmatic conditions. The beauty of ginkgo is that it interferes with a protein in the blood responsible for causing spasms in bronchial tubes. For best results, take 60 to 240 milligrams of standardized ginkgo extract a day. If you exceed that amount, you risk diarrhea, irritability, and restlessness.

Shrink symptoms with evening primrose. Evening primrose oil may reduce the airway inflammation associated with asthma. Experts recommend two 500-milligram capsules of evening primrose oil three times a day.

Let coleus forskohlii relax bronchial muscles. Coleus forskohlii has been shown in studies to be as effective as prescription asthma drugs, without causing the shakiness, tremors, and other unwanted side effects associated with those medications. Keep asthma under control by swallowing 50 milligrams two or three times a day. Look for standardized extracts of this herb that contain 18 percent forskolin, the substance experts believe is the active ingredient in this herb.

Tone down swelling with licorice. To reduce inflammation, select a standardized licorice-root product (such as capsules) that contains 12 percent glycyrrhizin. Take two capsules three times daily.

Athlete's Foot

Just because it's called athlete's foot doesn't mean you can only get itchy, peeling, cracked feet in the gym. You can pick up your own case by

WOMAN TO WOMAN
Her Asthma Is under Control

During a 10-year time period, Kerry Taylor, 48, of Northampton, Massachusetts, was hospitalized more than 10 times for asthma, usually for more than a week at a time. Her asthma got so bad that at one point, she completely stopped socializing for fear of an attack. Here's how herbs changed her asthma and her life.

I didn't develop asthma until I was in my twenties. It started as a cough, and although it bothered me, I just put up with it.

In my early thirties, I had the worst bout of my life. My lungs felt as if they were closing down—as if someone had poured a sticky, thick sludge in them—and I was suffocating. I finally saw a doctor and began taking corticosteroids to reduce inflammation.

The medication didn't make me any better, so I checked into a hospital. Still nothing seemed to work. At one point, I sat up for three days straight because if I lay down, I couldn't breathe. I attached a pillow to the hospital tray over the bed so I could lean forward and try to get some rest that way, but I never got more than a few minutes of sleep. There just wasn't enough air.

I eventually got over that episode, but soon trips to the hospital became a common occurrence. More important,

walking barefoot around swimming pools, locker rooms, even your own bathroom—if someone else with the infection has been there before you.

Athlete's foot occurs when a fungus sets up house in the damp skin between your toes and on the bottom and sides of your feet. There, it quickly goes to work, causing all kinds of mischief to the skin of your feet. Ditch the itch and soothe your toes with herbal remedies that some natural healers say not only help to oust the fungal infection but also make you less susceptible to future invasions.

frequent attacks were ruining my personal life. I couldn't go to the movies or eat out because if somebody walked by with a cigarette, I'd be gasping for breath in no time.

My world grew smaller, and my relationships were suffering. The first time you're in the hospital, everyone is there encouraging you. But by the 8th, 9th, or 10th time, they don't always show up, and when they do, they're sort of nervous around you. Even my best friend was worried to be around me.

In my late thirties, I moved to a small city where I met a wonderful doctor. Knowing that I already had an interest in herbal healing, he encouraged me to investigate herbs and other alternatives to supplement my asthma medications. To my surprise, they actually helped! Herbs such as astragalus, which strengthen the immune system, made me less sensitive to triggers and prevented me from getting colds and bronchitis. Since then, I've added some other herbs to my repertoire. Whenever I feel a respiratory illness coming on, I take elderberry, which prevents the virus from invading the respiratory tract cells. I treat my cough with wild cherry and hyssop cough syrups. To help keep my sinuses clear, I use eucalyptus essential oil in the shower and bath.

Using my medication and these herbs has given me a handle on my asthma. I can now go to the movies, visit friends, walk through the fields. It changed my whole life.

Mix an antifungal soak. Tea tree essential oil helps fight athlete's foot fungus. Put it to work in a footbath: Once a day, mix five to seven drops of tea tree oil into four ounces of warm water in a tub big enough to hold your feet. If you need more liquid to cover the affected area, you can double this recipe. Soak your feet for 20 minutes to ease the itching and soothe cracked skin and infected nails. Then dry your feet thoroughly with a clean towel and put on clean cotton socks.

Follow up with a calendula salve. After you've used an antifungal soak for three days, add calendula cream or salve to your routine. The petals of this sunny, yellow and orange flower have been used in traditional skin-healing remedies. Look for calendula cream or salve in a health food store or through mail order. Apply after soaking and drying your feet. You can use the calendula salve up to three times a day.

Control the itch all day with ginger—and more. Fight the itch of athlete's foot with a light, fragrant foot powder made with ginger and tea tree oil. Both herbs have antiseptic and antifungal properties, so they fight the fungus and can help control bacterial infections in skin already inflamed by athlete's foot.

Combine one-half cup of powdered arrowroot, one-half cup of cosmetic clay, and two tablespoons of powdered ginger; cover the mixture and shake it. Add 20 drops of tea tree essential oil and shake it again. Store it in a covered, dark glass jar in a cool, dry place. Apply it as needed to your feet. This powder will also help control moisture, making your feet a less hospitable place for athlete's foot to breed.

Bad Breath

Are friends constantly offering you mints? Is your loyal beagle backpedaling when you bend to offer a smooch? A mouthful of germs could be giving you bad breath.

The culprit behind offensive mouth fumes may be a nighttime's worth of germs that multiply gleefully before you can brush and gargle in the morning. Aromatic food and drink, such as garlic-laden pasta, raw onions, or coffee may also leave a lingering scent that contributes to bad breath. If chronic bad breath hounds you for weeks, see your doctor or dentist. She can check for serious health conditions such as diabetes, liver or kidney problems, a bad tooth, or infected gums.

Of course, regular brushing and flossing are the first steps to take against garden-variety halitosis. Add to this daily dental routine the following herbal mouth fresheners for naturally sweet breath.

Munch some parsley. To quell common food-related mouth odor, chew parsley after meals. This green sprig contains chlorophyll, a well-known breath deodorizer. Or skip the sprigs and swallow parsley capsules such as BreathAsure (containing parsley and sunflower oil).

Crunch cardamom. This popular Arabian spice is full of cineole, a powerful antiseptic that kills bad-breath bacteria. You can buy whole cardamom pods at health food stores and some supermarkets. Rejuvenate your breath by splitting the pods and chewing on a few of the seeds found inside. Discreetly spit out the seeds when you're finished.

Concoct a spicy mouthwash. Homemade cinnamon mouthwash curbs unpleasant mouth odor as well as or better than some brand-name mouth rinses. Combine 10½ tablespoons of ground cinnamon with 1¼ cups of apple-cider vinegar in a bottle with a tight-fitting lid. Let it sit for two weeks, shaking twice daily (morning and night). Then strain this so-

---

GETTING THE STING OUT

If you get bitten or stung by an insect out in your backyard or while hiking, you can quickly ease the pain and swelling by using some local plants, says Angela Stengler, N.D., a naturopathic physician and herbal author in Oceanside, California.

1. Pick a handful of fresh plantain or chickweed leaves. When searching for plantains, look for a low-to-the-ground plant with egg-shaped, smooth leaves that are three to eight inches long. The small white flowers grow elongated spikes, which protrude from the middle of the plant. The plantain grows from March until October. Chickweed plants have freely branching stems that root at the plant's base. Smooth, oval leaves grow along the stems, and small

Plantain
Look for plantain growing wild along roadsides and other marginal areas. It may even be in your own backyard. Its ribbed leaves grow from the center of the plant and surround seed stalks that look like miniature cattails.

lution through cheesecloth or a coffee filter and store it in a clean glass or plastic bottle. To use it, swish and gargle for one minute to fight bad breath.

white flowers cluster at the stem tips. Chickweed plants form a thick mat on the ground. They grow under cool, wet conditions in early spring. Make certain there is no dirt on the leaves you pick. Also make sure that there are no neighboring poison ivy plants that may have spread their oils to the healing plants.

2. Rub the leaves together in your hands until they are juicy.

3. Place the wet leaves on the bite or sting for 15 to 30 minutes.

4. If a gauze pad is available, place it over the wet leaves and fasten it with a larger piece of rolled gauze.

Chickweed

Look for chickweed growing under trees (especially oak trees) and in other shady places. Its tiny star-shaped white flowers grow on a tangled stem along with pairs of small, succulent light-green leaves.

Try a minty anti-halitosis tea. When muck mouth overpowers you (or others), kill the germs that cause bad breath with peppermint tea. Drink a cup whenever your breath needs

freshening. The aromatic oil in this mint acts as a potent antiseptic.

Bites and Stings

You know the buzz. And you certainly know the sting. When mosquitoes bite or bees sting, their attacks can cause redness, fire-hot pain, unrelenting itching, swelling, and, sometimes, skin infection.

The annoying winged creatures fall into two categories: blood-suckers and stingers. Mosquitoes, fleas, black flies, deer flies, and itsy-bitsy mites want to suck your blood. Bees, wasps, yellow jackets, and velvet ants defend themselves by jabbing you with the tiny, poisoned harpoons in their butts. (Of these, only the honeybee leaves her stinger behind in your skin, along with a sac of venom.) If you're stung by a bee, first safely remove the stinger and sac by scraping them away with your thumbnail or a credit card.

One note of caution: People allergic to insect venom can develop life-threatening reactions. If you have difficulty breathing or develop hives on your arms, legs, or torso, call your local emergency medical number or head to the nearest hospital pronto.

Otherwise, try these simple herbal soothers for fast relief from the pain, itch, swelling, and infection.

Stop pain and itching with peppermint. Get fast, long-lasting relief by rubbing a tiny droplet of peppermint essential oil into the bull's-eye center of bites and stings. Peppermint essential oil has been used traditionally as an antiseptic and local anesthetic. It cools the area, reducing itching and pain. Thoroughly wash your hands after application so that you won't irritate your eyes.

Dab on calendula. This herb encourages tissue healing and acts as a natural, infection-fighting antiseptic. Make a calendula tea, using about one tablespoon of the dried herb per cup of boiling water. Let it steep five minutes, then strain and let it cool. Dip a cotton ball into the calendula tea and dab it on bites or stings four or five times daily until the skin has healed.

Soothe inflammation with echinacea. For stubborn bug bites that stay swollen, ease the inflammation with an echinacea poultice. For a small bite, combine one teaspoon of echinacea tincture and one teaspoon of water with enough bentonite clay to create a thick paste. The clay can be purchased in some health food stores or herb specialty shops. (You can double this recipe for larger or multiple bites.) Dab the mixture on the bite and cover it with an adhesive strip bandage. Reapply the paste and change the dressing twice a day.

A large German study demonstrated that echinacea, when used topically, regenerates tissue, reduces swelling, and spurs the body's immune system into action.

As an alternative, drink 60 drops of echinacea tincture mixed in one-quarter cup of warm water three times a day for up to two weeks.

Breastfeeding

As natural as breastfeeding your baby is, sometimes nature needs a little nudge. You want to make sure your breasts have enough milk for your newborn—not too little or too much. And being a good mom means being good to yourself as well as your baby. You may need relief from sore, cracked, or even bleeding nipples after nursing.

If you think your milk production could use a boost, discuss trying the gentle, safe herbal remedies mentioned below with your doctor.

While taking any medication—natural or otherwise—is usually prohibited during breastfeeding, some herbalists recommend a class of botanicals known as galactagogues for nursing mothers. These herbs have been recognized as milk enhancers for hundreds, if not thousands, of years.

Build your milk supply with herbal tea. Daily stress can prevent you from producing enough milk to satisfy your baby. You can restore calmness and help boost your milk production by sipping a multi-herbal blend.

Combine one part each of oatstraw and chamomile and one-half part each of lavender and nettle. Add a pinch of fennel seed for each cup of tea you make. Steep one teaspoon of this blend in a cup of boiling water for 15 minutes, then strain and sip. Research suggests that lavender, chamomile, and oatstraw are calming agents, while nettle and fennel seem to promote lactation.

Try a simple fennel brew. Pungent fennel seed displays mild estrogen-like properties, and for centuries, women have used it to promote milk production. Try it yourself with a tasty fennel tea. Use two teaspoons of crushed seeds per cup of boiling water, steep it for at least five minutes, strain, and sip. Have up to three cups each day.

Soothe sore nipples with aloe. Your baby may go gangbusters when it comes time to nurse, but your nipples may pay the price. Heal the nipple area and ease pain with aloe vera gel. Snip a leaf from an aloe plant, slit it open lengthwise, and scrape out the cool, clear gel. Spread it on your nipples. It's best to use the gel after breastfeeding—and be sure to wash it off thoroughly before your next feeding. Aloe's bitterness is not something your baby would enjoy.

Breast Pain

How are your breasts feeling? Uncomfortable? Swollen? Achy? Estrogen, a female hormone, may be to blame. When estrogen levels are high—usually just before and during menstruation—one or both breasts may swell and become achy, tender, even lumpy. Estrogen stimulates fluid retention in breast tissues.

Levels of discomfort vary. One woman may feel mild tenderness, another excruciating pain. Doctors say that breast pain is very common and usually not a cause for alarm. Most of the time, your menstrual cycle is the cause.

You can reduce discomfort by cutting back on or eliminating caffeine-rich foods and drinks, including coffee, black teas, colas, and chocolates. All contain substances that may contribute to pain. Also, limit your intake of animal fats, which seem to raise estrogen levels. Plan your meals around organic whole grains, vegetables, and fruits, which help to keep your hormone levels in balance.

Now, you're ready for step two. Herbalists favor these botanicals to correct hormonal imbalances and assist your body in processing hormones efficiently.

Tame the pain with black cohosh. Studies demonstrate that this pain-relieving herb also acts as a mild sedative and reduces swelling in tender breasts. Take a dropperful of black cohosh tincture (also called an extract) in tea, juice, or warm water three or four times a day for several months until the symptoms dissipate.

Curb the ache with evening primrose. If you've eliminated caffeine from your diet but still experience painful and swollen breasts before your menstrual period arrives, natural healers recommend evening primrose oil, an effective anti-inflammatory herb. Take one or two 500-milligram capsules two or three times a day.

Reduce swelling with an herbal combo. Ease breast tenderness and pain caused by swollen lymph nodes by mixing a simple herbal combination. Combine equal amounts of tinctures of cleavers, milk thistle, rosemary, and sarsaparilla. Drink one-quarter to one-half tea-

spoon of this mix three to five times a day, in water, juice, or tea, until the lumps start to go away. These herbs help to move fluids through your body's lymphatic system and prevent them from pooling in lymph nodes. They also help balance hormone levels.

BEARBERRY

Good for: chronic bladder problems, including urinary tract infections

Bronchitis

Call bronchitis the never-quit cough. That deep, raspy, painful hacking can last for weeks, thanks to upper respiratory infections that inflame and irritate the airways leading to your lungs.

If you have bronchitis, your lungs are probably congested with mucus, creating an ideal breeding ground for infection. It's important to reduce your risk of lung infections, including pneumonia, by getting this mucus up and out. If your cough gets worse or you feel weak, tired, short of breath, or feverish, it is important to go to the doctor to rule out pneumonia. The only way to know for sure is to have a chest x-ray. If you haven't reached that stage yet, follow these herbal strategies to calm a hard-to-shake cough and clear congested lungs.

Inhale eucalyptus vapors. Commission E, a group of scientists that advises the German government about herbal medicine, says that eucalyptus essential oil is an effective expectorant for loosening phlegm. Inhale eucalyptus vapors to treat bronchitis and its persistent cough. One way is to create your own personal steam bath.

Place several cups of water in a tea kettle and bring it to a boil. Carefully pour the steaming water into a bowl, and add several drops of eucalyptus essential oil. Drape a large towel over your head and lean over the bowl about 12 inches or so, close enough to feel the steam without burning yourself. Breathe deeply, inhaling the eucalyptus vapors as they waft toward your nostrils.

Soothe the mucous membranes with mullein. Relieve inflamed mucous membranes and help remove mucus from the lungs with mullein tea. Steep two teaspoons of this dried herb in a cup of just-boiled water for about 10 minutes. Strain and drink. Have up to three cups a day. As a bonus, mullein also reduces swollen glands, which often accompany bronchitis.

Rub in spicy relief. Reduce lung congestion with this easy-to-assemble herbal vapor rub recommended by natural healers. In a glass bottle, combine one-quarter teaspoon eucalyptus essential oil, one-eighth teaspoon peppermint essential oil, one-eighth teaspoon thyme essential oil, and one-quarter cup olive oil. Shake the oils to mix evenly. Gently massage the mixture onto your chest and throat as needed.

Calm the cough with plantain. English plantain has a worldwide reputation as an effective cough suppressant and bacteria fighter. Make a hot tea, using one teaspoon of dried plantain per cup of water. Steep until cool, then drink as needed.

Bruises

The coffee table. The door frame. The desk. Ouch! Sometimes it seems as if they're just waiting for an innocent shin, hip, or thigh to stumble their way. And when one finally stops you, it leaves a colorful, ugly, painful bruise.

Bruises happen when blood vessels break beneath the surface of your skin and leak small amounts of blood, which can cause pain and swelling. A woman bruises more easily as she gets older because collagen—the connective tissue that cushions skin—breaks down, leaving blood vessels more vulnerable to bumps and collisions. Certain medications, including blood thinners like aspirin, also increase your risk of bruising.

Most bruises heal on their own within a few weeks. You can chart the healing process as the bruise changes colors: first reddish blue, then purplish black, then yellowish green. But you don't have to wait weeks for improvement. Hasten the healing process and ease the pain and unsightliness with these botanical treatments.

Reach for arnica. Also called mountain daisy, arnica contains an active ingredient, helenalin, that clinical studies show relieves pain and reduces swelling from bruises. Stop using it if your skin becomes red, itchy, or inflamed after applying the arnica.

Call on calendula. The ancient Greeks swore by these bright yellow and orange flowers when it came to mending bruises. To craft an herbal poultice, soak one tablespoon of dried calendula flowers in an equal amount of warm water until they're rehydrated—they should look more like fresh flowers. Or if fresh calendula is available, simply crush some petals. Then place the petals directly on the bruise, keeping the herb in place for three to four hours with an adhesive strip. Use gauze and tape for a larger area. The sooner you apply the poultice, the better the chance you'll avert severe swelling, pain, and discoloration.

Chill the black-and-blues with parsley ice cubes. Have this icy herbal remedy on hand in the freezer so that you can put the brakes on swelling quickly next time you're nursing a new bruise. Put a handful of parsley and one-quarter cup of water in a blender, then blend until slushy. Fill ice cube trays halfway with this mixture and freeze. When you need relief, wrap a parsley ice cube in gauze or a thin cloth and place it directly on the bruised site for 15 to 20 minutes. Parsley is a traditional bruise-mender, and the ice will help relieve or prevent swelling.

Stock up on flower-powered herbal ice. Place one teaspoon of chamomile flowers and one teaspoon of lavender flowers into a pan. Add one cup of boiling water, cover the pan, and let the mixture steep for about 15 minutes. Strain out the herbs. Freeze the tea mixture in an ice cube tray. When the tray is frozen solid, pop out the cubes and store them in a plastic freezer bag. When the next bruise occurs, wrap a thin cloth around an herbal ice cube and apply it to the bruise. Ice it for 10 to 20 minutes; repeat every two hours.

In addition to the inflammation-soothing powers of the ice, the chamomile and lavender in these bruise-cubes discourage swelling and promote faster healing.

Burns and Scalds

Every year, 1½ million people accidentally burn themselves at home. Although it's hard to imagine a more painful wound, most burns and scalds are minor and can be treated safely at home without the need for a trip to the emergency room.

Be prepared for these household emergencies by stocking up on the best appropriate herbal remedies.

Be Ready for Burns!

Even a small burn can hit you hard in the pain department. Here are some important do's and don'ts from experts on how to minimize pain and speed healing of first- and second-degree burns.

- ✦ DON'T ice a burn. Ice is too cold and might cause even more damage to the skin. Instead, soothe a burn by applying cool water.

- ✦ DON'T slather on butter. When the outer layers of your skin are gone, you're more vulnerable to infection, and any food product, including butter, can be loaded with bacteria.

- ✦ DON'T bandage the burn tightly. Instead, cover it with a loose, clean dressing so the burned area and any affected joints can move. By allowing movement in the area, you'll boost circulation to the area and speed healing.

- ✦ DON'T mess with the blister. If a blister appears on burned skin, your body has created its own bandage to protect itself.

- ✦ DO fill up on fluids, which will keep your skin well-hydrated and help improve its ability to heal.

- ✦ DO eat plenty of protein and vitamin C. Both nutrients will help rebuild collagen, one of the building blocks of skin tissue, and speed healing.

- ✦ DO seek immediate medical care if the burn is extremely tender, painful, swollen, and blistered; if it has pus, yellowish drainage, or a yellowish crust; if the area around the burn looks red or feels hot; or if you have signs of a fever.

- ✦ DO try this herbal remedy for minor burns recommended by herbalist Rosemary Gladstar, director of the Sage Mountain Herbal Education Center in East Barre, Vermont, and author of *Herbal Healing for Women*.

Blend one or two drops each of peppermint and lavender essential oils with one tablespoon of honey. Gently dab the mixture on the affected burn site. Loosely cover with a gauze wrap; leave the wrap on for a few hours or overnight. Reapply as needed until the skin heals. Lavender and peppermint first cool the burn and then take away the pain. Honey acts as a disinfectant, blocking germs from entering the wound.

Then, the next time you accidentally finger-hug a hot cup of tea or brush against a curling iron, you'll be ready to minimize pain and skin damage—quickly.

Before applying any herbal treatment, immediately run cool water over the burned area. This cools the skin and relieves pain. Then reach for these herbal soothers and skin healers.

Treat it on-the-spot with aloe. Simply snap off one of the spiky outer leaves of an aloe plant and slit it open lengthwise. Squeeze the transparent-colored gel out of the leaf and onto burned skin.

The clear, cooling gel inside this common, easy-growing plant offers protection against pain, reduces swelling, and dilates capillaries, which brings more blood—and more of the body's own team of skin menders—to burn-damaged skin. Aloe also contains vitamins C and E and zinc—nutrients that speed wound healing.

Reduce scarring with two skin-friendly herbs. Calendula and comfrey have earned reputations as skin menders. Researchers believe that triterpenes in calendula spur the growth of new cells and that allantoin in comfrey hastens tissue repair. Apply a salve containing calendula and comfrey to minor burns. Never use comfrey on deep burns or on burns that show signs of infection like redness, puffiness, or oozing. It can heal surface skin so quickly that it may trap the infection underneath.

Cool the burn with a botanical bath. Fill your tub with cool water, then head for the kitchen and prepare this herbal burn fighter.

Bring one quart of water to a boil, then turn the heat off and pour in one-quarter cup each of comfrey leaves, plantain leaves, and calendula flowers. Stir in three drops of lavender essential oil and one cup of colloidal oatmeal (a finely powdered oatmeal available at drugstores) or regular oatmeal milled in a coffee grinder. Steep this mixture for 20 minutes. Strain. Pour it into your cool bath and soak.

BURDOCK
Good for: psoriasis, eczema, and acne

Caffeine Addiction

Yes, coffee is an herb. But herbalists consider it the Jekyll and Hyde of the botanical world. Made from the roasted and ground seeds of the *Coffea arabica* plant, coffee—in moderation—perks you up, improves your reflexes, and helps you concentrate. It can also send your pulse and heartbeat racing, elevate blood pressure, trigger menopausal hot flashes, and bring on jitters and headaches. And there is some controversial evidence that consuming too much caffeine can aggravate the painful, but harmless, breast lumps sometimes referred to by doctors as fibrocystic breast disease.

Although coffee is the first item to come to mind when we think of caffeine, its jolt is also found in teas, colas, and chocolate. How much is safe? As a benchmark, experts recommend no more than a 5-ounce cup or two of coffee a day—or one 8-ounce cup of tea or one 12-ounce can of soda.

Many of us consume much more than that. If you're ready to give up caffeine but you worry about losing that energizing zip—or if you're concerned about the headaches that can come with caffeine withdrawal—relax. Herbs can ease withdrawal symptoms. The real key to kicking the caffeine habit is to make a gradual shift—by replacing caffeinated beverages with a drink that's flavorful and boosts your energy levels in a healthier way. Here's how.

Sip green tea. Start weaning yourself away from coffee by drinking green tea instead. This herbal tea contains 40 to 100 milligrams of caffeine per cup (the amount increases with steeping time)—about as much as coffee. But unlike coffee, green tea also contains polyphenols and catechins, compounds that protect your heart by lowering cholesterol. These substances also provide some cancer-protecting qualities and act as powerful antioxidants.

Brew a natural energy booster. Once you have successfully trimmed back your daily dose of caffeine, try this energizing tonic. Blend equal parts of chicory root, dandelion root, and milk thistle seed. Use one tablespoon of this mix per cup of boiling water. Steep at least 5 minutes (10 to 15 is better). Chicory, dandelion, and milk thistle are thought by herbalists to stimulate your liver. They also assist your body in fighting stress.

Canker Sores

What is tiny, stays out of sight, and instantly ruins your enjoyment of even the finest gourmet meal? No, not your pager going off in your pocket. A canker sore.

Also called mouth ulcers, these recurrent, crater-shaped lesions can pop up almost anywhere on your tongue, inside your lips, or on the mucous membranes that line your cheeks.

What triggers a canker sore attack? Stress, nutritional deficiencies, tongue biting, bacteria, and highly acidic or salty foods are among the most common agents. But no matter what the cause, aggravate a canker sore with even the smallest slosh of vinegary salad dressing, and for the next few moments, pain will be the only thing you know.

Fortunately, most canker sores heal themselves within a week or so. You can shorten their natural course and keep yourself comfortable with these herbal healing strategies.

Rinse with echinacea. A little bit of echinacea goes a long way in healing canker sores, thanks to active constituents that boost the immune system. Try this mouth rinse: Add a dropperful or two of echinacea tincture to a glass of water. Two or three times a day, swish this rinse around in your mouth, then spit it out.

Try tea tree oil and water. Treat your canker sore naturally with a mouth rinse made from tea tree essential oil. This volatile oil from an Australian tree possesses antiseptic qualities. Simply add a few drops to a cup of water. Look for a tea tree oil product that contains 15 percent or less of cineole to avoid irritating your skin.

Go for grapefruit power. Biting into a section of tart, acidic grapefruit would be torturous for anyone saddled with a canker sore. Yet, in the form of grapefruit seed extract, this fruit provides welcome relief. Grapefruit's sour powers outmuscle bacterial infections in your mouth.

Quell mouth pain by dabbing some grapefruit seed extract directly on the canker sore several times daily. As an added boost, add five drops to a glass of water and swish the solution around in your mouth three times a day.

Cervical Changes and Genital Warts

Name the most common sexually transmitted diseases these days, and you're sure to mention AIDS—and perhaps herpes, syphilis, or gonorrhea. But don't overlook the human papillomavirus (HPV), a virus that causes genital warts, changes in cervical cells, and, if left untreated, even cervical cancer—often without detectable symptoms.

This highly contagious virus can infiltrate skin on the genitals or anus, or invade the vaginal wall or the outer surface of the cervix. Transmitted through sexual contact with an infected partner, internal HPV infection offers no telltale signs—it can only be detected by a Pap test. There, the presence of HPV shows up as abnormal changes in cervical cells—changes that make these cells resemble cancer cells. Although cervical changes (also called cervical dysplasia) are not cancerous, this condition must be taken very seriously because it can develop into cancer if not treated in time.

By contrast, you may see or feel external genital warts, also caused by HPV. If these swollen bumps appear on your genitals or anus, they may itch. But if they appear inside your cervix, genital warts are flat and symptom-free—even though they can be caused by the most virulent strains of HPV.

You can reduce your risk of contracting HPV by using condoms during sexual intercourse. It's also important to have an annual gynecological exam, including a Pap test, to detect the presence of warts or cervical changes. If HPV is discovered, get prompt treatment; never try to treat genital warts or cervical changes on your own.

Natural treatments can help tremendously. If you would like to go the natural route, work with an experienced physician who is well-versed in herbal medicine. Herbal therapy, managed by a good doctor, can help prevent the progression of the disease, reverse cervical changes, and prevent recurrence. A doctor will also know when you should have a biopsy or even have precancerous cells removed. Along with doctor-supervised natural therapies, you can take steps at home to soothe discomfort and boost your immune system during treatment. Here are a few herbal strategies to consider.

Bolster immunity with garlic and a saintly herb. Garlic and St. John's wort are among the leading immune-enhancing herbs that can tackle an invading virus. Experts recommend taking two to four capsules of garlic daily and four dropperfuls of St. John's wort tincture in the morning and evening every other day.

Bathe in oatmeal. Soothe wart-related genital itching with Aveeno bath treatment. You can purchase it in any drugstore. This product contains a finely powdered oatmeal called colloidal oatmeal, known to ease itching. It also won't clog your bathtub drain.

Smooth on an herbal soother. Apply a cream or salve containing calendula, plantain leaf, aloe, or chamomile to your vulva morning and evenings as needed. These herbal creams stop the irritation, redness, and itching of genital warts. Select creams that do not contain perfumes or essential oils that might irritate tender mucous membranes. These creams can be purchased in health food strores or through mail order.

CALENDULA
Good for: reducing topical inflammation and fighting infections

Chapped Lips

Every day, indoors and out, the climate attacks our lips. Baked by the sun's rays and dried out by heat, air-conditioning, and wintry winds, they can chap, crack, redden, and blister. Licking your lips to restore moisture only makes matters worse.

Your lips are fragile: While a pigment called melanin protects the rest of the skin on your body from the elements, your lips lack this weather guard. So, it's up to you to provide some dependable protection against assault. Try these herbal helpers for moist, pain-free lips that can stand up to the elements, indoors or out.

Moisturize with castor oil. Purchase a

small bottle of castor oil at the drugstore and tuck it into your purse. Dab a few drops on your lips to soothe the sting caused by cracking. This inexpensive oil coats your lips and offers a thick lacquer of shine.

Stir in skin-friendly eucalyptus. For really chapped and sore lips, add 10 drops of eucalyptus essential oil to a two-ounce bottle of castor oil. Dab on lips as needed. Eucalyptus gives the castor oil a skin-healing boost.

Look for a healing balm. Herbalists recommend the herbs lavender, calendula, plantain, nettle, chamomile, and comfrey to soothe chapped lips and promote healing. Look for a ready-made, all-natural lip balm in your local health food store that contains one or more of these healing herbs. The best balms are made with olive oil and beeswax, which herbalists recommend to moisturize and protect lips.

Colds and Flu

When will it finally happen? We've been waiting, and waiting, and waiting. When will they discover the cure for the common cold? We need that magic bullet, and we need it now!

Don't lose hope. We may not have a cure yet, but that doesn't mean you're stuck with all those nasty symptoms. Herbal therapies have unique powers to boost your immune system so that it can better fight off the hundreds of different cold and flu viruses just waiting to invade your body and reproduce by the billions in your nose, throat, and lungs.

These invaders strike most often in winter.

THE HERBAL KITCHEN
Stinging Nettle Tea

"If I had to choose one herb to hang out with, it would be stinging nettle," declares herbalist Rosemary Gladstar, director of the Sage Mountain Herbal Education Center in East Barre, Vermont, and author of *Herbal Healing for Women*.

Gladstar says that nettle leaves make a delicious tea and contain a variety of nutrients, especially vitamin A, vitamin C, calcium, magnesium, potassium, zinc, and iron. So the next time you have a sore throat, upset stomach, cold, cough, or congestion, try Gladstar's spinachy-tasting stinging nettle tea recipe as a nice complement to other decongesting remedies.

- 1 teaspoon dried stinging nettle leaves, or 2 teaspoons fresh stinging nettle leaves
- 1 cup water
- 1 teaspoon honey (optional)

If fresh nettle is available, wear gloves when picking young, tender, light green nettle leaves from their stems to avoid the plant's stinging hairs. Discard the stems. Thoroughly wash the leaves and put them in a pan of boiling water. Cover with a lid. Boil for 20 minutes. Cooking renders the plant stingless. Strain out the nettle, and if you prefer, sweeten the tea with the honey. To make one quart, use 4 to 6 teaspoons of fresh nettle or half as much dried nettle.

During this peak season, we're more likely to come in contact with nasty viruses because we spend more time indoors with other folks who may already be nursing a respiratory or digestive ailment. Then, simply touching something—a doorknob, telephone, or anything that has been handled, sneezed at, or coughed on by a sick person within the previous 24 hours—heightens your own risk.

Beyond boosting immunity, botanical strategies can also help knock out a cold or flu in its early stages, and they can minimize symptoms at any point, bringing you relief. Here's how to take advantage of their powers.

Stockpile echinacea. At the first sign of illness, take a dose of echinacea, long hailed among Native Americans as the classic cold-and-flu warrior. Scientists say echinacea activates the production of two proteins in your body—interferon and properdin—that battle viruses.

Follow the package dosage directions for echinacea tinctures, capsules, or tea. But be sure to take it often: every hour or two for the first day, then three times a day until your symptoms have subsided. Continue taking echinacea for about three more days once you're feeling well. One note: If you use echinacea tincture "straight" (without water), you may notice a slight numbness in your mouth immediately after taking a dose. This sensation is harmless and short-lived, and it's a sign that you have genuine echinacea.

Heap on the garlic. Crushed or mashed, garlic is an antiviral herb that helps take the punch out of a cold. If you're worried about bad breath, take enteric-coated garlic capsules in 300-milligram dosages three times a day for as long as cold symptoms last. Then, breathe a sweet-smelling sigh of relief. If you don't mind garlic breath, eat several raw cloves a day—chopped and added to salads, soups, or entrées—until your symptoms subside.

Try a berry good virus fighter. Elderberry contains two compounds that prevent flu viruses from invading respiratory tract cells. Studies have shown that flu sufferers who used an elder-

REAL-LIFE SCENARIO

What's a Germaphobe to Do?

Helen is 39 and loves her job in medical sales. She meets a lot of great people on sales calls to hospitals and doctors' offices, and she enjoys socializing with them. As much as she enjoys her work, being exposed to a "sick" environment and spending a lot of time around people who deal with the sick has made Helen kind of phobic about germs. So she fortifies herself against them: She washes her hands incessantly and takes megadoses of "protective" nutrients, such as vitamins C and E, beta-carotene, and the trace mineral selenium. She is also experimenting with quercetin, coenzyme Q_{10} (CoQ_{10}), and dimethyl sulfoxide (DMSO). On top of that, she drinks several cups of echinacea tea a day—she wants to stop a cold before it starts. Still, she's worried she may not be protected enough and wonders: What else is out there?

Helen may not be catching any colds these days, but she does appear to have a mild case of mysophobia—that's a fancy word for an irrational fear of germs.

It's normal to worry about staying healthy when everyone around you is sniffling and sneezing, but she has become completely preoccupied with trying to avoid contamination. She should discuss her phobia with her doctor, who may recommend meditation or other stress-reduction methods to help her deal with her anxiety.

Helen also needs to rethink her supplement strategy. She's right about one thing—taking certain vitamins, minerals, and herbs *can* help her natural defenses ward off a cold or the flu. But taking megadoses of supplements is not as protec-

berry product showed significant relief of fever, muscle aches, and other symptoms within 24 hours. Read the label for proper dosage amounts.

Soothe aches and nausea with ginger tea. Ginger is well-regarded by herbalists for its stomach-soothing and ache-relieving abilities. For nausea and muscle aches, drink a cup of ginger tea up to four times a day. Simmer one tive as Helen may think. Too much of even the most beneficial nutrients can cause side effects. High doses of vitamin C, for example, can cause diarrhea. Excessive beta-carotene can turn her skin yellow. And DMSO—a solvent usually used on the skin to aid the absorption of certain drugs—may be harmful when taken orally.

Instead of swallowing a smorgasbord of supplements every day, Helen would do better to take a multivitamin that provides the FDA's recommended daily values of her essential nutrients. She should also concentrate more on eating a healthy diet, getting plenty of rest, and exercising regularly, all of which will help reduce the effects of stress and boost her immune system.

Her herbal strategy needs a bit of reworking as well. Drinking several cups of echinacea tea a day provides her with little protection because the herb actually loses its immune-boosting power when taken too often. Instead, Helen could drink just one cup of echinacea tea on weekdays and take the weekends off. She might also add a daily dose of another herbal immune-system booster, astragulus.

Helen is already following the best strategy to prevent catching a cold—washing her hands. But there's no need to wash them incessantly. That will leave her hands dry and chapped. One good suds and rinse after each of Helen's sales visit is probably enough to rid her of any virus-causing germs.

Expert consulted
Jennifer Brett, N.D.
Naturopathic physician
Stratford, Connecticut

teaspoon grated fresh ginger and one cup water in a covered pot for 10 minutes. Then strain and sip.

Congestion

Breathe in . . . breathe out. You draw air in and out of your lungs automatically 23,000 times a day. Each inhalation brings in the fresh oxygen that every cell in your body needs. But it's also an open invitation to airborne dust, pollen, and tobacco smoke as well as cold and flu viruses, all of which can leave you feeling stuffed up.

Dust and smoke act like sandpaper, scraping and irritating the delicate membranes in your nose and sinuses. Cold and flu viruses can also irritate these membranes, causing them to swell. This blocks sinus passages so that they can't drain. The result? Congestion—that all-stopped-up, can't-breathe feeling.

The next time you are saddled with a stuffy nose and want relief, turn to these safe herbal remedies, which can offer comfort without side effects.

Reduce stuffiness with herbal steam. The moist steam rising from a hot herbal tea can help break up nasal and chest congestion caused by colds, flu, smoke, or allergies. Select pungent herbs like peppermint, ginger, yarrow, thyme, or lemon verbena. Add a handful to a pot of boiling water. Then turn off the heat and place the pot on a trivet on the kitchen counter. Cover your head with a large towel and lean over the pan. Keep your head about 12 inches above the pot. Slowly breathe in the vapors alternately through your nose and mouth for about 10 minutes. You can bring your face closer as the steam cools.

The hot vapors from these herbs help liquefy mucus, fight germs, and open passageways in the nose, sinuses, and chest.

Unclog gingerly. To reduce inflammation and open clogged nasal passages, natural healers rely on ginger tea. In part because of its rich zinc content, some herbal healers say ginger may do for clogged noses what Drāno does for clogged kitchen drains. Finely chop a one-quarter-inch slice of fresh ginger and add it to one cup of water. Boil gently in a covered pan for 10 to 15 minutes. Strain and add a squeeze of lemon or a spoonful of honey if desired.

Lay on the onion. To help break up chest congestion, dice two onions and place the pieces in a pan. Cook gently with a little oil until the onion bits are transparent. Cool, then lay the pieces across your chest. Place plastic wrap over the onions (use a piece that fully covers the onions). Put a warm towel or warm water bottle wrapped in a cloth on top of the plastic wrap. Leave the onions on your chest for about 30 minutes.

The secret behind this old-fashioned remedy are the essential oils in the onions. They're believed to help fight any infection related to the congestion. Onion also stimulates blood flow, say herbalists, which they believe helps your body break up congestion and move waste material away.

Constipation

Have trouble moving your bowels? You're not alone. Some 50 million Americans experience constipation each year. But are we all talking about the same problem? Some people define constipation as stools that are too hard. Others apply the "C-word" to stools that are infrequent, small, or difficult to pass. With all of those irregularities, cramping, bloating, and pain can make the picture even more complicated.

The truth is that if you were to ask around, you wouldn't be able to find one hard-and-fast description for constipation—or for bowel regularity. Some people average a bowel movement every day, while others seem to be on an every-three-days schedule. Notice what seems normal for you. Constipation is simply any deviation

from normal that makes your bowels more sluggish.

Women sometimes become constipated the week or so before their menstrual periods. Hormonal fluctuations can slow normal bowel activity, while premenstrual cravings for fatty, sugary foods may mean you're getting less of the fiber that helps your bowels operate optimally.

The best strategy for getting your bowels back on track is to adjust your eating plan. Consuming at least five servings of fruits and vegetables and two servings of whole grains, and drinking at least eight eight-ounce glasses of water per day will increase the bulk and water content of your stools, making their passage through your colon easier. Of course, to be on the safe side, you should see your doctor if you notice any sudden change in your bowel movements, including the size, color, consistency, or the presence of blood.

In addition to improving your diet, try the following herbs to gently coax your bowels back into action.

First, try flaxseed. Take a teaspoon of whole flaxseed, grind it in a coffee grinder, and stir it into an eight-ounce glass of water or juice. Sip one of these flax cocktails with each meal until constipation subsides. Flaxseed is rich in fiber and also contains substances that help balance hormones.

Prompt faster action with dandelion. This common "weed" contains bitter compounds that can help stimulate contractions of the colon and move stools along. It is also thought to stimulate bile flow. Herbalists recommend using one to three dropperfuls of dandelion root tincture in one-quarter cup of water. (A dropperful is about 15 drops.) Drink slowly, savoring each mouthful for about a minute.

Soften stubborn stools with licorice and prunes. When all else fails, call on the bowel-loosening team of licorice root and prunes.

Make a licorice-prune tea by simmering one-half teaspoon of licorice root in one-half cup of water for two minutes. Remove from the heat and steep for 15 minutes. Strain out the root and soak three stewed prunes in the tea for a few hours. Eat the prunes and drink the tea (have them cold or slightly warm) before going to bed to give stools a needed nudge. You should experience relief by morning.

Coughs

It's very hard to stop a cough. And for good reason, you shouldn't even try. Coughing is a natural reflex designed to expel excess mucus from your lungs.

Still, a cough may erupt at the most inopportune times—as you're ready to address your church committee, as you're sleeping at 2:00 A.M., or in the middle of a tender love scene at the movies. It could be a throat-tickling dry cough. Or a phlegm-raising, rattling cough. A cough that bursts forth like machine gun fire or a soft but insistent cough that just won't quit. In any case, a persistent cough can inflame your throat and even make your chest hurt.

For stubborn coughs that don't disappear after two weeks—or that bring up discolored phlegm (not clear or whitish)—see your doctor. Otherwise, try these natural ways to silence that hacking.

Summon horehound to the rescue. For aggravating coughs, suck on cough drops con-

WOMAN TO WOMAN

Herbs Help Mom-to-Be

Carol Gilmore, a 35-year-old researcher from Easton, Pennsylvania, loves being a first-time mother to 1-year-old Rachel. Careful not to take medications during her pregnancy, Carol sought help from her herbal-trained midwife when she developed chronic constipation midway through her pregnancy.

I have always had an interest in herbs. I take echinacea tincture at the first sign of a cold and drink slippery elm herbal tea blend when I feel a sore throat coming on. I prefer taking the natural approach whenever possible.

At the end of my first trimester, I began to feel discomfort whenever I tried to have a bowel movement. I was no longer regular. For about a month, the bowel movements were hard and dry, and they really hurt. At the same time, I was taking prenatal vitamins with folic acid to help prevent birth defects. I was also drinking at least 64 ounces of water a day. I needed help.

I talked to my midwife, Beverly Fleming, about my symptoms and asked what I could do safely and naturally to clear up my constipation. She recommended an herbal blend containing dandelion root tincture and orange peel tincture. On her instructions, I blended these herbal tinctures and took them about 10 minutes before each meal. She explained that dandelion stimulates the liver to release bile, which can have a laxative effect. Orange peel is a warming stimulant that builds digestive function.

It was miraculous how fast—and well—these herbs worked. I was very impressed at how something so simple and natural could have such a positive effect. There were no side effects and no dangerous chemicals in my body. At the end of my pregnancy, I delivered a healthy and beautiful little girl.

This herbal mix definitely worked for me. It's one I can rely on if I ever develop constipation again.

taining horehound, natural healers suggest. This herb acts as an antispasmodic, soothing muscle spasms that produce coughs, as well as a decongestant.

Give a cough the slip with slippery elm.
To calm a persistent cough and soothe your irritated throat, herbalists recommend slippery elm throat lozenges. Native Americans relied on this herb for cough relief because it contains large amounts of mucilage, which acts as a mild cough suppressant. Herbalists recommend taking slippery elm in throat lozenges instead of tea because the lozenges provide a steady stream of mucilage to coat your throat.

Call for tea thyme. Relax airway muscles and clear up congestion by drinking thyme tea three times a day for up to three days. Thyme acts as an expectorant and relieves bronchial spasms triggered by excessive coughing. To make the tea, pour six ounces of freshly boiled water over 1²/₃ teaspoons of fresh thyme leaves (or ½ to ²/₃ teaspoon dried thyme). Cover and steep for 10 minutes, then strain. Let the tea cool before drinking it. After three days, stop this remedy and see your doctor if your coughing and irritated throat do not improve.

Clear up congestion with elecampane.
For coughing accompanied by thick congestion, herbalists suggest elecampane root tea. Pour one cup of cold water over one teaspoon of chopped elecampane root in a saucepan. Simmer for about 20 minutes, strain, then drink the warm tea. Have up to three cups of this tea a day while you have a cough. Elecampane root expels mucus and dries out mucous membranes. Plus, it contains mucilage, so it soothes your irritated throat. This herb is bitter-tasting, so you may need to add some honey to sweeten it a bit.

CHAMOMILE
Good for: soothing an irritated stomach and easing muscle spasms

Crow's-Feet

If you follow twin sisters, one a lifeguard, the other a bookkeeper, from the beginning of their careers to their 30th birthdays, "sister sun" will have more crow's-feet—those tiny lines radiating from the corners of the eyes—than will her sister. Why? Sun exposure.

First, sun glare plays a role. Squint long and often enough, and the temporary wrinkle patterns that form at the corners of your eyes will eventually become permanent. At the same time, skin exposed to sunlight for years loses its elasticity more quickly than protected skin and becomes drier. Sunlight destroys collagen, the protein that makes up the fibrous portion of your skin. With less collagen, wrinkles happen more easily.

Dermatologists recommend protecting your skin by wearing a sunscreen daily to block some of the sun's powerful rays. They also agree that you'll get fewer crow's-feet if you never smoke, squint, or tan your face.

Herbalists suggest these natural steps to avoid crow's-feet, or at least to prevent existing ones from deepening.

Remoisturize with cocoa. Keep the area around your eyes moist by applying skin lotions and cosmetics daily that are enriched with cocoa butter. Cocoa contains emollients that help prevent dryness while moisturizing and softening the skin. Coconut oil is a similar tropical emollient that offers the same benefits.

Pat on papaya. To loosen and remove old, sun-wrinkled cells on the skin's surface, make a homemade facial peel using papaya and fresh pineapple juice. The peel will reveal a layer of smooth, fresher-looking skin.

Purchase a papaya, an orange-green skinned tropical fruit, in the supermarket's produce section. It doesn't have to be ripe to work. At home, mash one-quarter cup of pulp. To enhance its skin-peeling properties, add one teaspoon of fresh pineapple juice to the mashed pulp. Apply this mixture to the wrinkled skin around your eyes. Be careful not to get the pulp in your eyes. (If you do, rinse immediately with cool water.)

You can also spread it on your entire face and neck. Leave the pulp on your skin for 10 to 15 minutes, then rinse with lukewarm water. It may sting slightly, but that's a sign that it's working. Repeat twice a week.

Usher in new skin with rose hips. Strong rose hip tea also works as a mild facial peel. The ascorbic acid in this herb peels away the upper layers of skin cells.

To make a rose hip peel, put one tablespoon of dried rose hips in one-half cup of boiling water. Steep for 15 minutes, then cool. Using your fingers, pat the cooled tea on the skin over your crow's-feet. Leave it on for 5 minutes, then rinse with tepid water. Finish the treatment by applying a light application of olive oil to moisturize the skin.

Cuts and Scrapes

Women are as prone to cuts and scrapes as their kids are. Slip on loose gravel and scrape a knee. Break a glass in the sink while washing dishes and slice a fingertip. Slip with the razor and scrape your shin.

Happily, your skin is prepared for these everyday emergencies. After an injury, your body's natural repair team quickly arrives at the scene to protect against infection and rebuild damaged cell layers. You can boost your body's innate healing powers by following some commonsense rules about caring for injured skin, and by choosing skin-friendly botanicals to help protect and mend everyday wounds.

How do you tell if your cut is more than a minor mishap? If the cut is large (more than one-half-inch long) or deep into the yellow, fatty layer of your skin, you need to see a doctor for stitches. Stitches help the cut heal faster and reduce your chance of scarring. You may need an antibiotic if the cut area is red, tender, or oozing pus, or if you have a fever.

For a minor cut or scrape, begin by cleaning out any dirt to reduce the risk of infection. Doctors suggest cleaning cuts and scrapes three times a day. Plain old soap and water works well, or you can try one of the following herbal washes to fight bacteria and swelling, protect sensitive, unhealed skin, and promote the birth of healthy new skin cells.

Prepare antiseptic herbs in advance. Get ready for the next cut or scrape by making this easy herbal antiseptic formula ahead of time. Mix one-half ounce each of the following tinctures (sometimes labeled as extracts): calendula, echinacea, Oregon grape root, and St. John's wort.

Store this mixture in a two-ounce dark glass bottle with a dropper in the lid. Mark the date on the bottle. This homemade first-aid tincture has a shelf life of about a year. When the need arises to clean a cut or scrape, dilute equal parts of the antiseptic mixture and sterile water (such as distilled water or filtered tap water).

Cleanse with myrrh. You can ease the pain of cuts and scrapes and fight infection with myrrh. This biblical botanical—a gift to the infant Jesus from one of the Three Wise Men—has been used for centuries as an astringent that prompts healing. Myrrh is a reddish brown resin that flows from the bark of a species of shrubs and small trees in Africa and southwestern Asia. Herbalists recommend dissolving one teaspoon of myrrh powder in one cup of warm water. Then use that liquid mix to wash out a cut right away.

Double up on the calendula. To promote healing and help clean up any residual debris caught beneath the skin, herbalists suggest calendula, used two ways. First, mix 25 drops of calendula tincture in four ounces of sterile water (available in most drugstores) and apply directly on the wound as needed. Then apply calendula ointment directly to the wound or dab some on a bandage and cover.

In the late 1800s, American cowboys used calendula to stop bleeding and heal bullet wounds. Researchers have found that this herb can also decrease swelling and spur growth of new skin cells.

Quell pain with St. John's wort. When scrapes cause pain, an infused oil of St. John's wort works better than aspirin, say some alternative medicine experts. Dip a cotton swab in the oil and apply directly to the cut.

COMFREY
Good for: reducing inflammation associated with bruises, sprains, and dislocations (topical application only)

Dandruff

Those annoying white flakes that shower down from your scalp onto the shoulders of your black sweater are more than an inconvenience. They're skin cells on the move.

In dandruff-free hair, new skin cells migrate to the surface of the scalp and shed without notice every 21 days. Dandruff results when these cells reach the surface in half the time. As a result, cells build up on your scalp in clumps before they're shed. When they do shed, they look like a snow flurry in your hair and on your clothing.

Oily hair and yeast infections of the scalp also prompt your head to shed dead skin cells in large clumps. Seasonal changes that dry out your scalp only make matters worse.

If dandruff makes your scalp red and very itchy and persists despite at-home treatment, see your doctor. You may need treatment for a fungal infection or for seborrheic dermatitis, an inflammation of the oil glands. For mild dandruff, natural healers suggest botanical remedies that work on the scalp itself as well as remedies that are taken internally. Combined, they help control itching and flaking.

Cleanse from the inside with burdock. Some herbalists believe that dandruff is a sign of an unhealthy liver, a signal that this vital organ isn't processing waste material from the blood effectively. They say you can attack dandruff from the inside out by improving the liver and cleansing your blood with burdock tea.

Prepare burdock tea with one to two teaspoons of root per cup of boiling water. Fresh grated root is best, but it is available for harvesting only from late spring through early fall. Dried, organic burdock roots are more readily available year-round from local health food stores. Boil these roots for 15 to 20 minutes, then strain the tea and drink up to three cups a day. You should see fewer flakes within a month.

Vanquish flakes with an herbal rinse. Stop itching and slow the buildup of white scalp flakes by rinsing your hair with this anti-dandruff formula. Take a handful each of dried nettle tops, dried calendula flowers, and dried rosemary and place these herbs in a two-quart glass jar. Cover the herbs with a quart of organic apple-cider vinegar. Close the jar and let it sit at least two weeks (ideally, one month) before straining.

Use one cup to rinse your hair after every shampoo and leave it in. If you find that it's too strong, you can use one to two tablespoons in one cup of water.

Boost scalp health with a witch hazel splash. Apple-cider vinegar mixed with skin-friendly herbs and witch hazel helps maintain the natural acid balance of your scalp, which will improve general scalp health. Create an herbal splash by infusing any combination of calendula, plantain, and comfrey in apple-cider vinegar.

Use a quart jar half-packed with dry herbs or fully packed with fresh herbs. Cover with the vinegar. Steep it for three to six weeks, then strain. For every three cups of vinegar, add one cup of distilled water and one-eighth cup of witch hazel. When you're ready to use it, mix about two tablespoons into a pint of water for an after-shampoo rinse.

Dental Health

How can you maintain a healthy, attractive smile? No news here. Brush and floss daily, and report faithfully for dental checkups twice a year.

You can further guard your smile by watching what you eat. Food and drinks loaded with sugar or acid (such as lemon juice) can cause plaque buildup, tooth-enamel erosion, cavities, and tooth decay. Beyond these basic strategies, however, herbalists offer botanical remedies for a host of common dental concerns.

Prevent plaque with bloodroot. To keep sticky dental plaque from adhering to your teeth, select toothpastes and mouthwashes that contain bloodroot. Studies have shown that dental-care products containing this herb can reduce plaque buildup on teeth within as little as eight days. Bloodroot contains sanguinarine, an alkaloid that chemically binds to dental plaque and keeps it from sticking to your teeth. Viadent, a popular mouthwash and toothpaste brand, contains bloodroot.

Trade diet soda for tea. To prevent cavities, switch your drink of choice from diet soda to herbal tea. A diet soda with a lemon twist may save you some calories, but it eats away at your tooth enamel. Green and black teas, by contrast, contain a generous amount of tooth-preserving fluoride. Four cups of tea per day—hot or cold—gives you all the fluoride you need.

Sweeten with sugar-free licorice. Need a bit of sweetness for your herbal tea? Licorice is not only a natural sugar-free sweetener but it also contains two tooth-protecting ingredients: glycyrrhizin, which kills bacteria, and indole, which prevents tooth decay. For a sweet taste, skip the table sugar and brew your green or black tea with a pinch of dried licorice root.

Depression

Every woman sings the blues from time to time. A relationship ends. A job promotion falls through. The last of your children leaves home to make her way in the big, wide world. That down-in-the-dumps feeling usually fades within a few days. But if it lingers for two weeks or more, it may be depression.

Research suggests that genes and biochemistry as well as personal history and recent life circumstances contribute to depression. It's an illness—not a character flaw—that can run in families. Hormonal changes just before menstruation and after pregnancy also appear to make some women more prone to feeling depressed. Certain prescription drugs and chronic illnesses trigger bouts of depression, too. Whatever the cause, the signs of depression can appear in every aspect of a woman's life. You may feel guilty, angry, or powerless. You may withdraw from others, overeat, lose your appetite, or find it difficult to sleep at night.

Martha loves to eat—especially chips, pretzels, and cheese crackers. She's quick to reach for a snack whenever she feels gloomy, often scarfing down a whole bag of tortilla chips after a tough day of teaching. But lately she seems to be down in the dumps all the time. And she's gaining weight. Martha recently saw an ad for low-fat chips listing St. John's wort as an ingredient. She read that this herb works like "natural Prozac" to relieve mild depression, so she stocked up on the snacks. Has Martha found the perfect answer to lifting her spirits while satisfying her mood-induced munching?

Probably not. Although some companies are jumping on the health bandwagon by adding herbs to foods, chances are the chips contain such small amounts of St. John's wort that they'll do little to improve Martha's mood. And even though the snacks are low in fat, they're probably loaded with empty calories— providing her with little nutrition and putting her at risk for even more weight gain.

Martha is right about one thing, though: St. John's wort *can* help to relieve mild depression—without the side effects of Prozac. That's why this "saintly" herb is the treatment of choice in Germany, where doctors prescribe one brand alone nearly 200,000 times per month to treat mild depression. Another potentially helpful herb, ginkgo, may also help to ward off Martha's blues by increasing blood flow to her brain and sharpening her ability to focus.

As for her mood-induced snacking, she'd be a lot better off replacing those chips with at least five daily servings of fruits and vegetables. These fiber-rich foods will fill her up, so she'll eat less, experience fewer cravings, and maybe even lose weight. And since her recent weight gain may be adding to her depression, trimming a few pounds may also help to lift her spirits.

Expert consulted
Dana Keaton, N.D.
Naturopathic physician
Head of the nutrition department
Southwest College of Naturopathic Medicine
Phoenix

Ranging from simple sadness or discouragement to suicidal despair, depression will affect one in four women over the course of their lifetimes.

Once you recognize that you're depressed, you can begin seeking relief. For severe depression (if, for example, you're having trouble functioning in your daily life or you have thoughts of suicide), see a doctor immediately.

Mild depression, on the other hand, may respond well to self-care with herbal remedies. Next time you get a case of the blues, give these botanical mood lifters a try.

Depend on nature's Prozac. Nature's top healer in the battle against depression is St. John's wort. Although this common, yellow-flowered plant has gained lots of attention in recent years, natural healers have actually relied upon it for thousands of years. And European researchers have concluded that St. John's wort works as well as standard antidepressants such as Prozac for treating mild to moderate levels of depression—without the side effects of drugs.

This herb appears to work in several ways at once: by normalizing levels of cortisol, a substance that helps your body deal with stress, and by activating the secretion of dopamine, a pleasure hormone.

St. John's wort comes in capsules, tinctures, or tea form. Check with your doctor or a qualified herbalist to select the best form for you.

If you choose capsules, slowly build the dosage to one 300-milligram capsule three times a day. For tinctures, take four dropperfuls in a little water in the morning and three in the evening. Some experts suggest looking for standardized St. John's wort products that contain 0.3 percent hypericin, one of the herb's active ingredients. Give this herb at least four to six weeks to take effect.

Soak in mood-lifting scents. For hundreds of years, healers have noted that the fragrance of certain herbs has the power to dispel a blue mood. Today, some herbalists and researchers believe that essential-oil fragrances may have an effect on the brain that is similar to that of antidepressants. Try it for yourself by adding this uplifting fragrance blend to your next bath: Combine two ounces of almond oil, 10 drops each of bergamot and petitgrain essential oils, 3 drops of rose geranium essential oil, and, if you'd like, 1 drop of neroli essential oil (it's expensive, so you can leave it out if you'd like). Pour the mixture into a tubful of warm water and soak.

By adding an additional two ounces of almond oil, you can turn this recipe into a fragrance to dab onto your wrists.

Sip the "happy herbs." Try a three-herb tea that can lift your spirits in three ways: It contains calcium-rich oatstraw, which strengthens the nervous system; lemon balm, which has a traditional reputation as the "gladdening herb"; and damiana, known in the Southwest as the happy herb. Damiana also is thought to balance hormone levels. Combine equal parts of all three, then use one teaspoon to one tablespoon per cup of boiling water. Steep five minutes, strain, and sip one to three cups a day.

Root out anger with dandelion. For depression that's more a case of unexpressed anger, down some dandelion root tea. It seems to help some women recognize and express withheld anger that can lead to feelings of numbness and depression, say some herbalists.

Use one tablespoon dandelion root per cup of boiling water, steep or simmer for 10 to 20 minutes, then strain and sip. Have two to three cups a day for best results.

Diabetes

When your body's fuel-delivery system is working right, carbohydrates smoothly convert into glucose, the body's chief source of energy. This simple sugar is then channeled through your bloodstream. It prompts your pancreas to secrete insulin, the hormone that ushers sugar into every cell in your body.

For women with diabetes, glucose can't enter cells efficiently. Either the pancreas doesn't produce enough insulin or cells resist the insulin's attempts to deliver sugar—or both happen at once. Uncontrolled, diabetes can cause serious, sometimes fatal, complications. Sugar can build up in your bloodstream, damaging your blood vessels, nerves, eyes, and kidneys. Wounds take longer to heal and circulation slows.

Doctors often prescribe insulin, to be taken either orally or by injection, depending on the type of diabetes you have. Type I diabetes requires daily insulin injections to maintain safe blood sugar levels. Non-insulin-dependent diabetes—Type II—can be controlled through a combination of diet, exercise, and oral medications that boost the effect of your body's insulin. Maintaining a healthy weight is also important.

DANDELION
Good for: stimulating the production of bile, which aids in the digestion of fat

While you should never stop taking insulin as prescribed by your physician, you can incorporate the following herbs into your daily routine to help regulate your blood sugar levels and possibly lessen the impact of diabetes. Be sure to talk with your doctor before adding these herbs to your treatment plan and continue monitoring your blood sugar levels carefully. Report any change to your doctor promptly.

Spice up your tea. Put a pinch or two each of bay leaf, cinnamon, cloves, and turmeric into a pot of black tea. Steep for 10 minutes. Pour over some ice in a glass and drink. Research shows that these spices help the body use insulin more efficiently.

Improve sugar stability with ginseng. Women with Type II diabetes may gain greater control of their blood sugar levels by taking ginseng. A Finnish study found that people with diabetes who took 200 milligrams of ginseng every day had stabler blood sugar levels.

Spoon up a special bean soup. To help maintain blood sugar at desired levels, try this fiber-fortified bean soup. In a large pan, bring two cups of water and one unpeeled onion (quartered) to a boil over medium heat. Add one 16-ounce can of kidney beans (rinsed and drained), one small diced carrot, one-half cup peanuts, one-half teaspoon fenugreek seeds, two bay leaves, four chopped garlic cloves, and a dash each of ground cinnamon, ground cloves, and turmeric.

Bring to a simmer, then cover and cook for 30 minutes. Remove the onion pieces with a slotted spoon, peeling off and discarding the skins. Lightly mash the onions with a fork and return to the saucepan. Discard the bay leaves. This recipe makes four servings.

Research has shown that beans, which are high in soluble fiber, help balance sugar levels. Onions, especially the skins, are rich in quercetin, which has been found to help with eye problems associated with diabetes. Fenu-greek contains six blood sugar–regulating compounds. Bay leaves may help your body use insulin more efficiently. And garlic may lower insulin resistance.

ECHINACEA
Good for: combating colds, flu, infections, slow-healing wounds, and inflamed skin conditions

Diarrhea

Diarrhea keeps you on the run—right to the bathroom. Those loose, watery stools are your body's way of saying "out with the bad."

Diagnosing diarrhea is easy. There's nothing subtle about the symptoms. Determining what triggers a sudden attack of the runs can be trickier. It could be a bacterial or viral infection, sudden stress, too much caffeine, or eating foods to which you're sensitive. All of these can irritate your intestines to the point of diarrhea.

Most diarrhea lasts no more than a few days, but during that time you could become dehydrated and lose valuable nutrients your body needs. And, of course, it's hard to maintain your day-to-day life when you're always dashing to the bathroom.

Before turning to any remedy—herbal or over-the-counter—scrutinize your eating habits and stress levels. People who consume high-fiber diets (lots of fruits, vegetables, and whole grains) and keep stress under control rarely have diarrhea. But if you need immediate relief, or if you still have minor diarrhea after altering your diet, try these herbal diarrhea stoppers. Of course, contact your doctor if diarrhea persists more than two days or if you see blood in your stool.

Call on cinnamon for emergency relief. Frequent bouts of diarrhea can lead to dehydration because your body is losing valuable fluids. To "dry up" bowels quickly, make some cinnamon tea. Cinnamon is a natural astringent that will curb the loss of fluids. To make the tea, mix one tablespoon of dried powdered cinnamon bark into one cup of hot water. Steep 10 to 15 minutes.

Curb the runs with blueberries. If you're on the road and unable to make a pot of healing herbal tea to stop diarrhea, natural healers suggest this take-anywhere remedy. Keep a bag of dried blueberries within easy reach. Chew and swallow three tablespoons for relief. Don't substitute fresh blueberries. They may actually cause diarrhea. Dried blueberries contain astringent tannins that reduce intestinal inflammation and help shield the stomach wall from toxins. The dried berries also contain absorbent pectins that can reduce fluid loss.

Soothe with slippery elm. Slippery elm bark is a popular diarrhea-fighter among herbalists because it contains slippery mucilage that soothes irritated intestines. Take a few spoonfuls of slippery elm powder, and blend in enough honey to create a thick dough. Roll the mixture into small balls. Finish by dusting the balls with a little more slippery elm powder. At the first sign of diarrhea, let a ball dissolve slowly in your mouth and repeat as necessary. Store the rest of the balls in a closed container in the refrigerator and use as needed. (To keep the balls indefinitely, dry them in a very low oven—just the pilot light will work—for a few hours or in the sun for a few days.)

Replenish lost nutrients with a multiherb tea. Important minerals, including potassium, chloride, and sodium, are washed from your body during bouts of diarrhea. These nutrients help your body regulate the flow of water across mucous membranes. You can restore them, herbalists say, by drinking a tea made with one or all of the following herbs: alfalfa, nettle, red raspberry leaves, and red clover. Use up to one tablespoon of dried herbs per cup of hot water. Steep about 15 minutes and strain the herbs. Then drink up to five cups a day until your symptoms retreat.

Dry and Sun-Damaged Hair

Dry hair looks dull and lifeless. It may stick straight out like the bristles on a broom, lay limply, or frizz up. Desert-dry tresses simply won't do your bidding—and you may be tempted, in frustration, to keep them hidden under a hat at all times.

What steals the shine and body? Blame the weather, which robs hair of moisture. But don't stop there. Our own primping also takes its toll, thanks to bleaching, coloring, straightening, perming, and using blow-dryers and curling irons.

Any of these can fry your crowning glory by damaging the outer layer of each hair shaft, called the cuticle. The cuticle consists of cells that overlap, sort of like shingles on a roof. Healthy cuticle cells lie flat, holding in moisture and reflecting light. This kind of hair feels healthy and looks shiny. But when cuticle cells get roughed up by intense heat or harsh chemicals, the hair shaft loses moisture and dulls.

These natural remedies should work beautifully to restore your hair's natural luster.

Make hair shimmer with essential oils. Add body and shine to dry and sun-damaged hair with this easy, deep-conditioning treatment using essential oils. Take one-quarter cup of olive, jojoba, or sweet almond oil and add 10 drops of lavender or rosemary essential oil. For thick, heavy hair, coconut oil works best. Wet your hair and rub in the oil mix until your hair is thoroughly coated. Cover with a shower cap and

THE HERBAL KITCHEN
Bath Salts

To add a little luxury to your bath routine, pamper yourself with homemade bath salts.

Tap water often contains calcium and magnesium, making it "hard." Hard water can leave your skin dull and rough. Bath salts counteract these minerals to silken and soften the water. They also help to remove body oils and perspiration.

Not only are bath salts relaxing and soothing but they're also easy to make. You need basic, easy-to-find ingredients, including borax, a natural mineral salt that is used as a laundry detergent. Try this simple recipe created by Mindy Green, a founding and professional member of the American Herbalists Guild, director of educational services for the Herb Research Foundation in Boulder, Colorado, and coauthor of *Aromatherapy: A Complete Guide to the Healing Art*.

   2   cups borax
   ½   cup sea salt
   ½   cup baking soda
   50   drops essential oil (about ½ teaspoon)

In a bowl, mix the borax, sea salt, and baking soda, then add the essential oil. Use ¼ to ½ cup bath salts per bath. For muscular aches and pains, add ½ cup of Epsom salts to the recipe. Store the mixture in a wide-mouth, dark-colored glass jar.

Essential oil suggestions: Use neroli, marjoram, or lavender for relaxing; rosemary, juniper, or eucalyptus for stimulation and muscle relaxing; or geranium or orange for stress relief.

a warm towel for 30 minutes. Then shampoo twice.

Concoct an herbal conditioner. Moisturize dry hair with an easy-to-make botanical conditioner. Combine one teaspoon of each of the following dried herbs: burdock root, calendula flowers, chamomile flowers, lavender flowers, and rosemary leaves. Pour one pint of freshly boiled water over the herbs. Allow them to steep for 30 minutes. Strain the mixture and add one tablespoon of vinegar. Wash your hair with a moisturizing shampoo (one that contains natural oils, glycerin, honey, or amino acids) and rinse. Then pour this herbal conditioner over your hair. Don't rinse.

Lubricate the ends, fragrantly. For dry, wispy hair, a few drops of sandalwood or rosemary essential oil works wonders on flyaway ends without leaving a greasy residue—and it smells great! Put two drops of either oil on your fingertips and massage it into the ends of your hair.

Moisturize from the inside out with evening primrose oil. Evening primrose oil is rich in essential fatty acids, which are vital to healthy hair and skin. Herbalists suggest taking one to three 250-milligram capsules of this herb one to three times a day. You can substitute flaxseed oil capsules, which also contain essential fatty acids.

Dry Skin

A woman's skin is vulnerable to all sorts of moisturize-robbing conditions, including sun, wind, and winter cold as well as the dry air in heated and air-conditioned rooms. These forces suppress oil production, leading to itchy, flaky skin.

You can fight dry-skin foes naturally. Start by drinking at least eight eight-ounce glasses of water daily to moisturize from the inside out.

Also make sure your diet includes oils high in monounsaturated fats such as olive and canola oil. In addition, wash with a water-soluble cleansing cream instead of soap. Most soaps dry out skin. And avoid facial toners that contain alcohol, another moisture stealer.

If your skin is still dry and flaky, try these gentle botanical remedies to restore a healthy, moist glow.

Sink into a tub of oats. If your entire body feels dry and irritated, an oatmeal bath can ditch the itch. The gentle cleansing power of oats seems tailor-made for dry skin. Their slippery quality soothes, moisturizes, and heals. To prepare an oatmeal bath, place one-half to one cup of old-fashioned rolled oats in a muslin bag or a handkerchief closed securely with a rubber band. Place the bag in the tub and run warm water. Don't pour oats out of the box into the tub or they'll clog the drain.

Alternately, you can soothe dry skin with Aveeno bath treatment, which is available in any drugstore. This product contains a finely powdered oatmeal called colloidal oatmeal, known to ease itching. It also won't clog your bathtub drain.

Switch to an herbal cleanser. If you have a dry complexion and need a soap substitute that won't rob moisture from your skin, natural healers recommend this easy-to-make botanical cleanser. In a bottle with a lid, blend two ounces aloe vera gel, one teaspoon of grapeseed oil, one teaspoon of glycerin, one-half teaspoon of grapefruit seed extract, eight drops of sandalwood essential oil, and four drops of rosemary essential oil. Shake well before each use. Apply this herbal cleanser with cotton balls, then rinse.

Blend a moisturizing mask. Soothe dry skin and protect against infection by applying this calendula-and-cream facial mask. Combine one-quarter cup of whipping cream, one-half teaspoon of olive oil, two tablespoons of mashed ripe avocado, and one teaspoon each of calendula petals and lavender flowers. Let this mixture sit for five minutes to allow the liquid to soak up the herbs. Then whip by hand or in a food processor. Slather the mask on clean skin and leave it in place for at least five minutes. The cream, oil, and avocado in this mask provide much-needed moisture, while the herbs add skin-healing properties. (If a ripe avocado is hard to find, skip it.)

Earaches

It aches, it throbs, it stabs you from the inside out, and you can't even rub it to make it feel better.

When you experience intense, lasting pain in your ear, something has usually gone awry deep in the Eustachian tube—the pencil-thin canal that runs from the back of your nasal passage to your ear.

Sometimes an invading virus or bacteria causes inflammation and fluid buildup in this narrow passageway. Colds, allergies, and sore throats can also bring on the kind of ear congestion that causes discomfort and muffled hearing.

Treating an earache is not always a do-it-yourself proposition. If it's sudden and intense or accompanied by dizziness, a fever above 101°F, or discharge from your ear, see your doctor at once. Severe ear infections can cause your eardrum to burst.

For less severe earaches, however, herbalists choose botanical remedies that can numb the pain as well as help your body knock out the infection-causing virus or bacteria. These herbs also strengthen your immune system to keep ear infections from making unwelcome comebacks.

Calm aches with St. John's wort oil. For extremely achy ears, St. John's wort helps stop pain by acting as an anti-inflammatory that soothes irritated nerves in the ear canal. This herb also helps fight viruses. Mix a solution of one-half St. John's wort infused oil and one-half mullein flower infused oil. (Mullein oil has antimicrobial properties.) You can purchase or order infused oils from your local health food store. Don't confuse them with essential oils. They're not the same. Put about three drops of this mix into the affected ear and cover with a cotton ball. Reapply the drops every six to eight hours, using a fresh cotton ball.

Gain relief with garlic. According to some herbalists, ear infections are no match for the antibiotic properties of garlic oil. For more ache-easing power, combine equal parts garlic and mullein flower infused oils. Put four drops of this mix into the achy ear and cover with a cotton ball. Reapply the drops every four to six hours as needed, using a fresh cotton ball each time.

Fight back with echinacea. Echinacea, also known as coneflower, may give your immune system a boost and battle infection. Steep one teaspoon of dried echinacea in a cup of boiling water for about 10 minutes. Strain and sip. Or add a dropperful of echinacea tincture to juice or tea. Drink either beverage three times a day until your earache goes away.

Eczema

Just what is that scaly rash that has been itching to drive you crazy lately? Is it serious? Will it ever go away? If it began as a reaction to stress, temperature extremes, or even scratchy clothing, then you may have eczema.

This skin condition often runs in families. Everything from emotional turmoil to extreme air temperatures to allergies can trigger an outbreak. So can extreme sensitivity to common foods like dairy products. In severe cases, eczema makes the skin thicken, blister, and crack, especially around the folds at your neck, elbows, and

knees. Anyone with a case this bad should see a doctor.

Eczema can be soothed by keeping your skin constantly moist. Have a moisturizer handy at work and at home. It's also smart to rule out possible foods that might be making matters worse. A simple diet change could bring relief. Then, rely on these herbal remedies to feel even better.

Pamper with slippery elm. Soothe itchy, inflamed skin rashes with an herbal paste. Mix slippery elm powder with enough water to form a thin paste. Apply the paste to the affected skin and leave it in place until it's dry—usually an hour or less. Rinse gently with water and pat your skin dry with a clean towel. Do this three times a day.

Slippery elm contains mucilage, which is known to moisturize, heal, and soothe skin.

Ditch the itch with evening primrose. You can soothe an eczema rash with evening primrose oil, an herb containing essential fatty acids that reduce inflammation. Take two to four 500-milligram capsules three times a day for best results.

Battle bacteria with goldenseal. For eczema that becomes infected, herbalists recommend goldenseal. Combine one part goldenseal tincture with three parts of warm water. Soak the mixture into a clean cloth and apply it to the rash for 15 to 20 minutes. Reapply this antimicrobial wash four or five times a day. Goldenseal contains berberine, a substance that fights bacterial infections, redness, and inflammation.

Endometriosis

Some women call it menstruation gone crazy. When you have endometriosis, heavy bleeding, sharp pain, and nausea can complicate your monthly periods. It can also inflict you with interrupted sleep, fatigue, depression, and infertility.

Endometriosis occurs when tissue from the lining of the uterus—the endometrium—migrates and grows on the ovaries, bowel, bladder, or other internal organs. This tissue expands, then sheds just as the normal uterine lining does during the course of the menstrual cycle. But since it's not in the right place, it causes pain and other problems instead of simply leaving the body as menstrual blood.

Medical experts don't know exactly why about 1 in every 10 American women develops endometriosis, but they theorize that an abundance of estrogen, a female hormone, can heighten the risk. Heredity and stress as well as environmental pollutants are also factors. Scientific evidence links endometriosis with a weakened immune system as well. There's no cure.

Conventional treatment calls for hormone-therapy medications, which suppress estrogen and lessen uncomfortable symptoms. In some cases, women have hysterectomies. You may be able to avoid these drastic measures by finding herbal treatments that alleviate most symptoms. After speaking with your natural health care professional, select herbs that reduce bleeding, swelling, muscle aches, cramping, and pain.

Ease pain with a nourishing tea. To fend off intense pain, herbalists often recommend this re-

REAL-LIFE SCENARIO

Painful Periods Have Her in a Quandary

Joanna woke up doubled over with menstrual cramp pain again this morning. And her sensitized vagina burned so badly whenever she wore tampons that she couldn't use them anymore. Her doctor diagnosed her problem as endometriosis and told her she may need a hysterectomy. She knows that left untreated, endometriosis could make her infertile. Both options scare her to no end. She's planning to get a second medical opinion, but a friend told her about a doctor who has been doing some amazing things with herbs. She is wondering: Should she be messing around with herbs for a condition that has so much at stake for her?

To find out exactly how serious Joanna's condition is, she needs a laparoscopy. This is an exploratory surgical procedure that will allow a doctor to see the extent of endometriosis in her abdomen.

Joanna might try using herbs for a brief period—no more than one to two months—to see if they bring relief. Then, if her doctor still feels that it's necessary, she can have the laparoscopy.

Herbal treatments can help a woman with endometriosis in two ways. First, they can lessen pain and cramping caused by the monthly buildup and shedding of blood in areas other than the uterus. Second, herbs can correct the hormonal imbalance that is thought to be at the root of most cases of endometriosis.

Valerian, peony, and tang kuei are often used for the pain and cramping, while chasteberry (also known as vitex), medicago, genistein (derived from soy), and a host of dietary supplements are commonly used to help balance hormones. Joanna should see a qualified naturopathic doctor who is skilled in handling women's health issues to get remedies that are tailored specifically to her.

Expert consulted
Jennifer Brett, N.D.
Naturopathic physician
Stratford, Connecticut

laxing, nourishing tea as the first step in a natural treatment plan for endometriosis. Combine equal parts of passionflower, damiana, and skullcap. Passionflower and skullcap ease pain; damiana relieves stress. Then add equal parts of alfalfa leaf, nettle, and raspberry leaf (which also balances hormones). All three of these herbs have a long history of relieving women's menstrual problems. For tea, steep one tablespoon of this blend in eight ounces of freshly boiled water for at least one hour in a covered container. Strain and sip. Have up to three cups of the tea a day.

Sip your way to improvement. For a front-line assault against the most intense symptoms of endometriosis, try this multi-herb blend tea that herbalists say balances hormones, curbs excessive bleeding, stops body-bending pain, and reduces inflammation.

Combine one teaspoon each of dried chasteberry, echinacea root, wild yam, and cramp bark with one-half teaspoon each of dried horsetail, raspberry leaf, and motherwort. Place these herbs in an uncovered pan with one quart of cold water and bring to a boil. Turn down the heat and simmer for 5 minutes. Remove from the heat, cover, and steep for 15 minutes. Strain out the herbs and drink two cups daily.

Make cramps disappear with a four-herb formula. For excruciating cramps, try a combination of Jamaican dogwood, kava kava, white willow bark, and valerian. Herbalists recommend taking 10 drops of each herb, in undiluted tincture form, two hours before bedtime and again right before you go to sleep. These herbs provide pain relief, stop muscle aches and spasms, and ease nervous tension.

If you try this tincture formula, don't exceed the recommended dose and use it only as needed, not on an ongoing basis. Since it can make you drowsy, use it only before bed or when you'll be home all day. Do not use it while driving.

Fatigue

Okay, so you're not the Energizer Bunny. Who is? In the real world, meeting the demands of job, family, home, and community leaves many of us exhausted. Instead of *going, going, going*, we wish we could just go to bed.

In surveys, 8 out of 10 women say they're tapped out from trying to do too much in too little time. Their fatigue comes not just from feeling overextended but also from feeling stressed. In response, we find ourselves reaching for quick pick-me-ups—another cup of coffee, another piece of chocolate, another snack cake from the vending machine. The trouble is that stimulants like caffeine and sugar may eventually leave you feeling even more exhausted.

The alternative? First, get a handle on why you're feeling so tired—and rule out underlying medical conditions. Ask yourself: How long have I been tired? Have I been under stress for a long time? What's making me so exhausted and why? Then take that information to your doctor.

If the checkup rules out medical conditions and determines that you're basically healthy, consider recharging with these herbal fatigue-blasting strategies.

Inhale peppermint for a quick lift. Rather than reaching for the coffeepot when you need a quick pick-me-up, grab a bottle of peppermint essential oil and inhale its stimulating scent. You can also put peppermint oil in a diffuser, a pump that blows the scent into the air. Place the diffuser in a convenient location, such as your desk at work or on the end table in your living room. Or you can just sprinkle a few drops of the essential oil into a small bowl of hot water. The steam will waft the scent through the air.

Grab Siberian ginseng for stamina. Siberian ginseng increases your resistance to all kinds of stress. Take one teaspoon of dried Siberian ginseng in a cup of boiling water, steep, strain, and then drink. It will take up to a month of continuous use before you'll notice any effects from using ginseng.

Be better with basil. Relieve mental fatigue with spicy basil essential oil. Add some droplets to a diffuser or sprinkle on a handkerchief and sniff when you feel tired.

Fever

To a certain extent, fever is your body's ally. When a virus or bacterium invades your body, your immune system literally turns up the heat to melt away infection or inflammation. This biological furnace enhances your body's ability to fend off these intruders.

Keeping that in mind, natural healers say you should let a fever run its course so that it can destroy infectious organisms and help you get well. If you suppress a fever too quickly, you hinder your immune system's attempt to defeat the invader. But if a fever goes above 103°F or lasts more than 24 hours, call your doctor. And if you do let a fever run its course, remember to drink plenty of fluids—otherwise, you may risk dehydration.

While over-the-counter medications may take the edge off of a fever, herbal treatments promote sweating so that it can run its course

WOMEN ASK WHY

If coffee can increase my stamina, get me through jet lag, and even ease my asthma, why is it so bad for me?

It's only bad for you if you drink too much of it. Try to keep your intake down to a cup a day. As with many medicinal botanicals, the herb itself isn't bad. It's how you use it that can damage your health. Some women simply drink too much.

Most people know that coffee contains caffeine, a substance that stimulates your nervous system. It also makes you more alert and can open up air passages, which is why coffee helps relieve jet lag and asthma. But some herbalists believe that it can rev up your adrenal glands as well. The adrenal glands, which produce a substance called epinephrine, are the pumps that fill you with energy and stamina. If you overstress them with coffee, they can "run dry."

Herbalists believe that the caffeine in coffee can be especially harmful to the health of women because:

- Caffeine can interfere with your menstrual cycle by inhibiting the breakdown of hormones.
- Caffeine aggravates the symptoms of premenstrual syndrome.
- Regular caffeine intake has been linked to decreased fertility.

You don't have to completely shun coffee, just cut back.

Expert consulted
Feather Jones
Professional member of the American
*   Herbalists Guild*
Director of the Rocky Mountain School
*   for Botanical Studies*
Boulder, Colorado

more quickly and effectively. Taking herbs may actually make you feel temporarily more feverish, but be patient. In the end, you'll likely feel a lot better.

Break a fever fast, with yarrow and more. To work up a sweat and break a fever, try this three-herb tea. Combine equal parts of dried elderflower, yarrow, and peppermint. Place 4½ teaspoons of this mix in a pint canning jar. Boil two cups of water and pour it into the jar over the herbs. Cover and let it steep for three to four hours. Strain and add honey to taste. This recipe makes two cups. After drinking a cup or two of this tea, you will start to sweat. Once that happens, you have had enough. Check with your naturopathic physician if you are unable to find some of these herbs.

Take nature's aspirin. For high fevers that cause body aches, turn to nature's original aspirin, willow bark. This herb contains salicin, the active ingredient in aspirin that reduces pain and swelling. For best results, swallow three or four 200-milligram capsules of willow bark extract a day while you have a fever. Make sure to buy a standardized formula that contains 15 percent salicin.

Replenish with natural ginger ale. If you're dehydrated, fresh, natural ginger ale will restore needed fluids and fight the germs that caused your fever. Try this easy-to-make natural ginger ale tea: In a saucepan, combine one teaspoon of thinly sliced fresh gingerroot (or one-half teaspoon ginger powder), one teaspoon of raspberry leaves, and three cups of water. Bring to a boil. Turn down the heat and simmer for 5 minutes. Remove from the heat and steep for 10 minutes. Strain out the herbs. Add one cup of carbonated water and one lemon slice just before you're ready to drink.

Gas

We would wish it away, if we could. But wishing won't do it. In fact, nothing will make it go away completely.

Most times, flatulence is nothing more than an annoyance. But sometimes, the sheer volume of gas in the intestines causes bloating, discomfort, and pain. Most of the gas you pass forms when undigested food wends its way into your large intestine and gets broken down by bacteria that live there. This process produces a foul-smelling mix of carbon dioxide, hydrogen, methane, and sulfur.

Gender doesn't play a role. Women pass gas an average of 12 times a day—the same as men. Eating habits, however, can be important. People who eat more protein than vegetables tend to have more flatulence because protein is a major source of sulfur, a gassy compound. Those with lactose intolerance, a condition in which they have trouble digesting milk sugar (lactose), also experience more gas. The artificial sweetener sorbitol triggers gas as well.

Although it's impossible to be flatulence-free, these herbs can help you control the intensity and frequency of untimely outbursts.

Put on the brakes with fennel. To ensure you're free of excess gas, chew one-half teaspoon fennel seeds. Fennel is a carminative, a substance that helps dissipate gas. It also helps correct digestive disturbances by relaxing muscle spasms.

Run out of gas with peppermint. Peppermint, another carminative, is a digestive-soother with a reputation for minimizing gas. For best results, pour one cup of just-boiled water over one tablespoon of dried peppermint leaves. Steep, covered, for 5 to 10 minutes, then strain and sip. Drink a cup of this tea three or four times daily.

Caution: Avoid drinking this tea if you have esophageal reflux.

Season with gas-banishing spices. If you enjoy eating beans or other gas-producing foods, you can tone down the tooting by seasoning your dishes with herbs from the mint and carrot families, herbalists suggest. Keep eating beans, which are an excellent source of high-quality protein, fiber, and other nutrients, but also reach into your spice rack for aniseed, basil, chamomile, cinnamon, garlic, ginger, lemon, onion, oregano, or rosemary—all of which are excellent carminatives.

EUCALYPTUS
Good for: bronchitis and throat inflammations

Gum Problems

Plaque turns white teeth a dirty shade of yellow, but this sticky film does its worst damage where you can't see it: below the gum line. In fact, plaque ranks as the top cause of gum disease, taking responsibility for about 80 percent of all dental problems in adults.

If you don't brush and floss daily, plaque—a soft, bacteria-packed film that forms on and between your teeth and under your gum line—becomes a rock-hard substance called tartar. Tartar irritates gums, causing them to swell, bleed, and become infected. These symptoms are signs of gingivitis, an early stage of gum disease.

Pregnant women are prone to gingivitis, especially during the first trimester. The rise in risk is related to rising levels of the female hormone estrogen during pregnancy, which seem to encourage certain types of plaque-forming bacteria to grow.

Ignore gingivitis, and your condition can worsen into periodontitis, causing gums to severely recede and teeth to loosen from your jawbone. But gum disease need not progress that far. Practicing mouth maintenance—brushing and flossing thoroughly and getting regular dental exams—will significantly safeguard the health of your gums.

You can also try these herbal treatments for additional gum-health insurance.

Herbalize your tooth brushing. In addition to your regular brushing and flossing routine, heal inflamed, diseased gums with goldenseal. Mix one tablespoon of goldenseal powder with enough water to form a paste. Then brush your teeth as you normally would. This bitter-tasting herb contains two alkaloids, hydrastine and berberine, that are potent antibiotics and inflammation fighters.

Fortify your water jet with echinacea. Fight off plaque and bacteria caused by food particles lodged in your teeth with a dental hygiene device (such as Water Pik) that uses a high-speed water jet. Then, bolster its healing powers by adding two to four drops of echinacea tincture to its water reservoir. Echinacea is acclaimed by herbalists as an effective oral antibacterial agent.

Drink chamomile after meals. If your gums are swollen and infected, drink a cup of chamomile tea after every meal. This herb helps to stop inflammation and kill germs, and it helps prevent gum disease. Infuse two teaspoons of dried chamomile in a cup of just-boiled water. Then let it steep for 5 to 10 minutes.

Sip or chew peppermint. Peppermint leaves help prevent gum disease by fighting the bacteria that cause tooth decay. To make a tea, steep two teaspoons of crushed fresh peppermint leaves in a cup of just-boiled water for 10 minutes. Then strain and sip. Or you can chew fresh mint leaves.

Why She Fears Fall

Marian woke up this morning with her head full of cotton and her nose running like a sieve. "Hay fever," she thought. **"Fall must be near." She could take antihistamines, but then she would be so groggy that she wouldn't be able to concentrate at work. Drinking stinging nettle tea, which she has heard herbalists often use to treat hay fever, only seems to make her symptoms worse. Her doctor has recommended allergy shots, but as far as she is concerned, needles are worse than allergies. What should she do?**

Marian shouldn't give up her quest to find a natural remedy for her hay fever. Her body didn't react well to nettle, but there are many other herbs that may help her to feel a whole lot better.

The first goal of herbal medicine is to prevent problems before they start. In the future, Marian should begin taking herbs four to six weeks before her symptoms usually appear. That will give her body time to prepare for the inevitable onslaught of allergens. Her best choices would be herbs that prevent the release of histamines, substances that cause the symptoms of an allergic reaction, into the bloodstream. Herbs that fall into this category include hawthorn, goldenrod, and dong quai (Chinese angelica).

Of course, that's for next year. For right now, Marian can take herbs that dissolve and dry up mucus and decrease the swelling in her nasal passages. These herbs include stoneroot, bayberry, and goldenrod.

If she continues having problems with bad reactions to herbs, she should consult a qualified professional who specializes in herbal healing to help her find herbs that won't cause difficulties. There's no reason that Marian can't get rid of her hay fever symptoms and avoid those needles she dreads.

Expert consulted
Irene Catania, N.D.
Naturopathic physician
Ho-Ho-Kus, New Jersey

Hay Fever

Hay doesn't cause it. And you don't get a fever when you have it. So what is hay fever, anyway?

Chalk up all that wheezing and sneezing to annoying airborne pollen. Hay fever occurs when your immune system goes a little haywire. Instead of limiting its assaults to bad boys, such as bacteria and viruses, it attacks harmless stuff like pollen, flooding your body with defensive chemicals called histamines. Unfortunately, this all-out response causes congestion, a runny nose, and itchy, watery eyes.

Some women find that pollen from flowering plants brings on hay fever's worst symptoms every year.

You can enjoy the changing seasons by turning to nature's best hay fever fighters.

Breathe relief with nettle. Prepare yourself for the approaching hay fever season by drinking nettle tea for at least one month ahead of time. This herb contains trace amounts of histamines, which stimulate your body to build immunity through its own natural antihistamine. To make a nettle tea, pour one cup of boiling water over one to three teaspoons of dried nettle. Steep for 10 to 15 minutes, then strain. Drink three cups a day. For best results, continue sipping the tea regularly during allergy season and for one month after it ends.

Make an herbal blend. For relief from sneezing and congestion and to bolster your immune system, combine one-half teaspoon each of tinctures of Siberian ginseng, nettle, elderflowers, and peppermint. Take half a dropperful at least five times daily, starting a few weeks before hay fever season begins. Siberian ginseng boosts immunity, and elderflowers help stop sneezing and relieve congestion. Peppermint helps clear congestion.

Headaches

Pounding . . . throbbing . . . pulsing. These are the adjectives women use to describe tension headaches, the most common type of head pain.

Muscle contractions characterize tension headaches. Pain usually starts in the muscles at the back of your head and neck, then it works its way to your forehead. Or you may simply feel a mild, steady throbbing just behind your eyes or in your temples. Stress is often the trigger, but marathon, eye-straining stints at your computer screen or sitting in a cramped position for a long time can also cause tension headaches.

Fortunately, these headaches usually disappear within a few hours, or even faster when you take aspirin or another over-the-counter pain reliever. But if aspirin isn't working, or if you're worried about its side effects, then consider these safe herbal alternatives to quiet the throbbing and relax the tension that brought on pain in the first place.

REAL-LIFE SCENARIO

Her Job Is a True Headache

Roxanne, age 40, was in perfect health—until she was promoted and transferred to a new area of the plant, where she now works as a chemical technician. First, she came down with a fierce cold that was the dickens to get rid of. Then came watery eyes, midday lethargy, and constant congestion. Finally, for the first time in her life, she developed headaches, which at present she blames on the demands of her new job, since she's headache-free on weekends. She hesitates seeing a doctor for fear he'll put her on powerful drugs, so a friend suggested she try an herbalist. Is this good advice?

Stress gets blamed for many headaches, but often it's not the cause. When it is the cause, the ache usually begins only after the stress has ended. In Roxanne's case, that would mean pain-free weekdays but long, throbbing weekends. In fact, she's experiencing just the opposite. So her trouble probably stems from something noxious in her work environment, not from job pressure.

Perhaps there's a smell in her new work space that's triggering her symptoms. That makes even more sense when you consider that Roxanne is a chemical technician and could work with any number of nasty substances.

Odors are common irritants. In fact, odors work on the body in a number of ways. Some trigger allergic reactions. In the same way that pollen or dust can cause the immune system to overreact, so can airborne chemicals. In other cases, the fumes that cause a smell directly irritate the mucous membranes of the eyes, nose, throat, and lungs.

Seeing an herbalist or naturopathic doctor is a reasonable thing for Roxanne to do. Consulting an occupational disease therapist would also be worthwhile, especially since Roxanne didn't have a history of headaches before changing jobs and workplaces.

Expert consulted
Jacqueline Jacques, N.D.
Naturopathic doctor
Portland, Oregon

Tame pain with feverfew or cramp bark. To stop the dull ache of a tension headache, take feverfew or cramp bark every hour for up to three hours. Follow the label directions on tincture or capsule bottles for the proper dosage. Feverfew contains salicylic acid, the active ingredient in aspirin, but in lower concentrations. Cramp bark has antispasmodic properties that herbalists say help relax tight muscles.

Reach for "herbal aspirin." For a pounding headache, try white willow, often nicknamed herbal aspirin. White willow contains salicin, an aspirin-like chemical that is easily absorbed by your digestive track. Unlike aspirin, however, willow bark probably won't irritate your stomach.

Soak away the pain with lemon balm and lavender. If your head throbs at night, a lukewarm herbal bath may bring relief. Add two tablespoons of dried lemon balm and two tablespoons of lavender flowers to a cup of just-boiled water. Steep 10 minutes, then strain. Pour this tea into a tub filled with lukewarm water. Ease in and soak for 20 minutes. Lavender and lemon balm are both known as relaxing herbs.

Mellow the ache with a calming herbal tea. For simple tension headaches, select one or more of these relaxing herbs: chamomile, linden flower, lemon balm, or passionflower. Brew a cup of tea using one teaspoon of your chosen dried herb or herb blend per cup of just-boiled water. Steep 5 to 10 minutes, strain, and sip. Between sips, take deep, relaxing breaths as your headache disappears.

WOMAN TO WOMAN
She Banished Her Headaches

In her 66 years, Eleanore Milardo has become all too well-acquainted with headaches. They plagued her from the time she was a young woman until they finally disappeared a few years ago. Then, just when she thought she was in the clear, the onset of menopause in her early fifties started the throbbing up again. This time, though, Eleanore fought back. Here is her story.

It's all pretty ironic. I'm a nurse trained to help heal people, but I couldn't even heal myself. From the time I was a teenager off and on throughout my life, I would frequently get these absolutely pounding headaches that lasted for 24 to 48 hours. I'd drag myself to work with them and feel sluggish and sick all day. My doctor diagnosed them as migraines.

In my thirties, I turned to natural remedies to ease the pain: I improved my diet, took vitamins, and tried a common herb for headaches called feverfew, all of which gave me some relief. Ten years later, even though I was still following the same lifestyle, I started having headache pain again.

I consulted my doctor, who quickly figured out what was wrong: A misaligned jaw joint was causing my headaches all this time. I got braces to straighten my teeth, had some other dental work done, and presto! No more headaches. Well, it wasn't quite that instantaneous, but you get the idea.

Heartburn

Maybe your heart isn't really on fire—but something inside you sure feels incendiary. That feeling comes from the sizzle that happens whenever stomach acid trespasses into the esophagus, the sensitive tube that connects your mouth to your stomach.

Heartburn usually strikes about an hour after a big meal or after you've eaten sugary or high-

So there I was, rejoicing that I was free. I didn't have to worry that tomorrow might bring another headache. I could live life like most other people do—working, grocery shopping, or doing whatever—without pain. But my freedom wasn't to last. When I started to go through menopause in my early fifties, I expected hot flashes and maybe some moodiness. Instead, I started suffering from headache pain again. And this time, I had no idea what was causing it. I hadn't yet realized it could be connected to menopause.

As a holistic nurse counselor and health food store owner, I read health information all the time. One day, I came across an article describing how hormone imbalances can cause headaches. Was this the crux of my problem? Excitement and hope bubbled up inside me.

I knew from selling herbs in my store that black cohosh was often used to balance hormones and help relieve menstrual problems. I began taking it every day. After about three weeks, I felt somewhat better. The headaches came less frequently and didn't last as long. By the time I had finished the bottle of capsules, the headaches disappeared completely.

That was 15 years ago. I continued taking black cohosh, but only when I felt I needed it, letting the frequency of headaches guide my usage. Now with menopause safely behind me, I can confidently say I have finally parted ways with headaches for good.

lems over time. If your heartburn is occurring three or four times a week for weeks at a time, it's time to see a doctor. Heartburn may be a symptom of something more serious. But if your heartburn is diagnosed as plain old . . . well . . . heartburn, your doctor may tell you to continue taking antacids. What can you do instead? Herbalists advise that you stay clear of fatty or sugary foods, cut back on coffee, and drink plenty of water. Then, try these herbal strategies.

Banish the burn with licorice. If you're prone to heartburn, take licorice before each meal. Deglycyrrhizinated licorice reduces the frequency of flare-ups by encouraging cells that line your stomach to produce mucus, which provides a "safety coating" that protects against your own highly acidic digestive juices. Take two 500-milligram tablets of deglycyrrhizinated licorice root 15 minutes before meals for best results. Make sure that you choose deglycyrrhizinated licorice, because it does not contain glycyrrhizin, a substance that can raise blood pressure.

Activate your digestion with turmeric. Season food with turmeric to keep your digestive juices flowing smoothly and food moving through your gastrointestinal tract without a hitch. If seasoning your food isn't enough to stop heartburn, take two or three turmeric capsules (for a total of one-half to one gram) before each meal.

Cool the fire with chamomile. Subdue heartburn pain, or prevent a new attack, with chamomile—a mild sedative that soothes mucous membranes. To make chamomile tea,

fat foods. That's because the cardiac sphincter, a gatekeeping muscle between your esophagus and stomach, gives way to pressure when you've eaten more than your body can handle. The muscle ring weakens and opens, allowing corrosive stomach acid to reflux, that is, to backflow and irritate the esophagus.

Some women rely on over-the-counter antacids to cool heartburn, but prolonged use of antacids can actually worsen esophageal prob-

THE HERBAL KITCHEN

Dill Tea

For more than 3,000 years, many cultures have turned to dill to ease digestive pain. In fact, the word *dill* comes from the Old Norse word *dilla*, meaning to lull or soothe. A cup of this dill tea, recommended by Shez Ward, an herbalist in Norfolk, England, and a member of the Royal Horticultural Society, will keep calm a stomach bothered by heartburn and indigestion.

    3   teaspoons dill seeds
    1   cup boiling water
        Honey

Using a spoon, bruise or pound the dill seeds until they break into small pieces. Put the seeds in a pot and cover them with the water. Put the lid on and let the tea steep for 30 minutes. Strain the tea, and add honey to taste.

vapor are among chamomile's active ingredients.

Hemorrhoids

In and around your anus and rectum are tiny, hardworking veins that expand during a bowel movement and shrink back to shape afterward. If you overtax them from prolonged sitting, straining while you're constipated, or lifting heavy objects, these veins surrender to pressure and can swell, ache, itch—or leave a harmless dab of blood on toilet paper after a bowel movement.

About half of all women develop hemorrhoids by age 50. Happily, most hemorrhoids come and go on their own within a few days. You can discourage these uncomfortable swellings by eating plenty of high-fiber foods and drinking lots of fluids. This combination of fiber and fluids helps bulk up the stool so it becomes softer and passes more easily through the rectum and anus.

Beyond these dietary tips, herbalists offer the following soothing botanical remedies for hemorrhoids.

Stop pain and swelling with witch hazel. If you experience painful, inflamed hemorrhoids, soak in a witch hazel sitz bath. Pour a pint of witch hazel into a tub filled with a couple inches of warm water. Sit in it for at least 15 minutes. Witch hazel acts as an astringent that shrinks swollen tissues and soothes pain.

Get your bowels moving with psyllium. For hemorrhoids brought on by the pushing and

add one tablespoon of whole dried chamomile flowers to one cup of hot water and steep for 15 minutes. Strain and drink daily. Some herbalists recommend that you keep the teapot and your cup covered so that the vapor can't escape. The volatile oils in the straining of constipation, turn to psyllium seed husks. Take 4 to 10 teaspoons of psyllium per day until symptoms vanish. Psyllium is a form of fiber that swells as it absorbs water in the stomach, adding bulk to stool and triggering muscle contractions that speed the waste along.

Soften stools with butternut. To soften stools and ease pain, herbalists suggest taking 20 to 30 drops of butternut tincture three times a day until your hemorrhoids disappear.

Herpes

Experts estimate that 50 to 80 percent of women have one of the two forms of *Herpes simplex*, the virus that leaves clusters of fluid-filled blisters around your mouth or your genitals. Only half of those exposed to the virus experience any symptoms, yet even symptom-free herpes-carriers can be contagious—and can unintentionally spread the virus to others.

If you do come in contact with herpes, the first symptoms can surface within seven days of contact. Your mouth or genitals—or both—may tingle, burn, and itch. Then, blisters appear, your skin reddens, and finally, the painful blisters burst. After that, herpes goes back into hiding until the next outbreak.

Like the common cold, herpes has yet to be conquered and cured, though antiviral medications may lessen the severity of an outbreak and increase the time between outbreaks. If you feel a burning or tingling in your genital area, followed by the eruption of small, red blisters that form a shallow ulcer, see your doctor or gynecologist. It goes without saying that you should nix sex if you or your partner has herpes blisters. While you can't stop this surly virus, you can subdue its symptoms and keep it dormant for as long as possible with these herbal strategies.

Bag herpes with black tea. To reduce pain and inflammation during a herpes attack, steep a tea bag filled with black tea for a few minutes in just enough boiling water to cover it. Let the bag cool and apply it directly to the herpes lesion. Black tea contains astringent tannins that may help dry out an outbreak.

Rely on lemon balm. Fight herpes with lemon balm, which contains compounds called polyphenols that prevent the virus from attaching to your body's cells, thus preventing the spread of infection.

Make a strong tea by steeping two to four teaspoons of dried lemon balm in a cup of just-boiled water. Steep, strain, and let the tea cool. Then, apply it directly to herpes blisters with a cotton ball several times a day.

Make a minty anti-herpes tea. Combine the virus-fighting power of lemon balm and other mint-family herbs in a tea that herbal experts say contains a dozen anti-herpes compounds. Fill a saucepan half-full with water and bring to a boil. Turn off the heat and add fresh lemon balm leaves until the pan is about three-quarters full. (If fresh lemon balm is not available, substitute one-quarter cup of dried lemon balm.) Then, add two parts each of dried oregano and self-heal and one part each of hyssop, rosemary, sage, and thyme. (The exact amounts don't matter, as long as there's twice as much oregano and self-heal.) Toss in a little licorice root as a sweetener and steep the mixture for 20 minutes before straining and drinking.

Keep the virus at bay with burdock and echinacea. To prevent recurrent outbreaks of herpes, create a gentle tonic using burdock root and echinacea. Prepare a very strong tea by using

FENNEL
Good for: easing painful gas and stimulating the appetite and digestion

one ounce by weight of each herb to one quart of water. Toss the dried herbs into a quart jar and fill it to the top with boiling water. Steep for four to eight hours, then strain. Drink one-half cup two to four times a day to limit outbreaks. Burdock acts as a mild antiviral agent and echinacea stimulates the immune system. Stop taking this infusion if you go three months with no outbreaks.

High Blood Pressure

Some women seem to live life inside a giant pressure cooker. There's pressure to do well on the job. Pressure to raise great kids. Pressure to have a good marriage, cover the monthly bills, maintain a home—and, of course, pressure to make time for a social life or community activities.

You know these pressures. They meet you head-on every day. But there's a type of pressure you may not even be aware of, and it can get the best of you: high blood pressure. Undetected and untreated, it can lead to two of America's top killers: heart disease and stroke.

High blood pressure occurs when circulating blood exerts too much pressure on artery walls, causing scarring, thickening, and hardening. Not only are arteries damaged, but your heart must pump harder to get the blood through. Stress, inactivity, a diet high in fats, and obesity all raise your risk for high blood pressure.

Only a blood pressure test can tell you whether or not your blood pressure is within safe ranges. For adult women, a blood pressure reading of 120/80 mm Hg (millimeters of mer-

cury) is considered normal, but a consistent reading of 140/90 mm Hg is considered high. Doctors recommend annual blood pressure screenings to be sure that yours stays within the safe ranges.

Fortunately, eating more fresh fruits and vegetables and getting regular physical activity can help control or prevent runaway blood pressure.

REAL-LIFE SCENARIO
She's Organic All the Way

Melanie, age 41, has followed an organic lifestyle since she was a teen. She's a vegetarian, shuns drugs at all costs, and only buys from health food stores. So she wasn't too pleased a few years ago when she started to struggle with heartburn and digestive upsets and developed borderline high blood pressure, which she blames on her irregular work hours and high-stress job as a waitress in a high-end Japanese restaurant. She first turned to peppermint tea, but it gave her heartburn, making her indigestion worse, not better. Then she read that licorice tea is good for heartburn and acid stomach—and it's been working just fine. The only problem is her blood pressure: It's still hovering above the safe limits of 140/90. Melanie's doctor insists that she go on blood pressure medication. She stubbornly refuses and is in search of a magical herb. Is there one out there?

Rather than going on a goose chase after an herbal magic bullet, Melanie should take some time to examine her lifestyle. Some simple changes might give her just the results she's looking for.

As a vegetarian, she's probably doing quite a few things right already, such as keeping her weight down; eating meals that are low in sodium, sugar, and saturated fat; and making sure her diet is high in fiber. It can be difficult to maintain a vegetarian diet that's nutritionally well-balanced, however, so she should make sure that she's getting enough calcium, magnesium, and vitamin C. All of these work together to keep high blood pressure in check.

Odd as it may sound, Melanie would also benefit from

eating lots of garlic and onions. Taking garlic in supplement form would be even better, since the concentration of allicin, the substance that fights hypertension, is higher. She should also consider taking a tablespoon of flaxseed oil and an herb called coleus forskohlii every day. Both of these have worked well in lowering some people's blood pressures.

Next, Melanie needs to take a close look at the herbs and supplements she uses. Some may actually contribute to raising her blood pressure. Licorice is a good example. Although licorice seems to have solved her problems with heartburn and upset stomach, it has a substance in it that can cause hypertension in some people. Instead, Melanie may want to try using deglycyrrhizinated licorice, or DGL for short. This is a special type of licorice extract that has the blood pressure–boosting substance removed. She might also think about switching from licorice to ginger, slippery elm bark, or chamomile, none of which will affect her blood pressure.

As for her heartburn and digestive problems, Melanie should investigate to find out if they stem from a food allergy or sensitivity. If they do, relief may be as easy as not eating peanuts, wheat, dairy products, or whatever food doesn't agree with her.

Finally, Melanie should get some help with stress management. Her heartburn, upset stomach, and high blood pressure could all be simply a result of a stressful lifestyle.

Expert consulted
Joan Haynes, N.D.
Naturopathic physician
Boise, Idaho

So can incorporating these herbal remedies into your life.

Jazz up your food with garlic. To lower blood pressure as well as cholesterol, natural healers suggest eating a clove of garlic daily. Studies have shown that a compound in garlic called allicin successfully deflates high blood pressure. Simply cook with garlic and use it in your salads. If you don't like its taste, take garlic in capsule form following the label directions.

Take lemon balm for relief. For high blood pressure triggered by stress, try a daily dose of lemon balm. Take five milliliters of lemon balm tincture twice a day for 12 weeks. Then recheck your blood pressure and continue taking as needed. Herbalists say lemon balm calms as it lifts your spirits, which can translate into lower blood-pressure readings.

Help your heart with hawthorn. To help strengthen your heart, reach for hawthorn, a centuries-old heart tonic. Make a tea using one teaspoon of dried hawthorn per cup of boiling water, and drink two cups per day. Or you can take five milliliters of hawthorn tincture twice a day. Hawthorn widens blood vessels, especially the coronary arteries, therefore lowering blood pressure.

High Cholesterol

You've no doubt heard that too much cholesterol in your blood—or in your diet—can contribute to heart disease. But did you know that cholesterol's not all bad? Your body needs some in order to function properly.

In fact, your body produces its own cholesterol to make adrenal and sex hormones. In addition, you need the good-guy, high-density lipoprotein (HDL) cholesterol around in order to help boot out the bad-guy, low-density lipoprotein (LDL) cholesterol, which clogs arteries.

Medical experts have set healthy levels for cholesterol at 60 milligrams per deciliter of blood for HDL and 130 milligrams per deciliter or less for LDL. Levels of LDLs above 130 heighten your risk for arteriosclerosis, a condition in which fatty deposits build up on the walls of your arteries. Blocked arteries lead to heart attacks and strokes.

Fortunately, you can lower your cholesterol with a low-fat diet and exercise. Beyond that, try these herbal helpers.

Go heavy on garlic. For a proven cholesterol-reducer that also lowers blood pressure, get garlic. Eat three to four fresh cloves a day in foods (minced and added to salads, soups, sauces, and stews) or take garlic capsules containing 3,000 to 4,000 micrograms of allicin (one of the active compounds in garlic) daily. More than 30 years of research shows that garlic lowers cholesterol and reduces heart disease risk. Some research suggests garlic also prevents the formation of blood clots that can block arteries.

Grab some guggul. Guggul is a gum resin closely related to myrrh. Some natural healers say it can raise HDL levels by as much as 20 percent and lower LDL levels by the same percentage.

Guggul creates more LDL receptors in the liver. They take more of the bad cholesterol out of your blood and excrete it through the feces before it can make fat deposits in your arteries.

Look for guggul products in standardized form. The recommended standardized dose is 25 milligrams three times a day. Take guggul until the lipid levels have normalized, and then reduce the dose to 25 milligrams once a day.

Sow health with fenugreek seed. Cut your LDL levels by consuming one to two tablespoons of ground fenugreek seeds three or four

REAL-LIFE SCENARIO

A Natural Solution to a Cholesterol Problem

Although she's under 40, Geraldine has been struggling with high levels of cholesterol and triglycerides for years. She knows that if she can't get them under control, her risk for heart disease—a problem that runs in her family—will escalate. When she reluctantly decided to take the cholesterol-lowering drug prescribed by her doctor, she found that it left her constipated. Her doctors switched her medicine, but she doesn't like the side effects of the new drug, either. She has read that a weird-sounding herb known as guggul can lower both triglycerides and cholesterol. She wants to give it a try but wonders how her doctor will react to it.

Geraldine is wise to take her high cholesterol level seriously, but she's right: Her doctor may not be enthusiastic about her using an herb he has never heard of instead of the medications he's used to prescribing.

So what can she do to help her case? First, Geraldine needs to educate herself as well as her doctor about the use of this herb. A little research would reveal that guggul has been used in India for thousands of years, and its uses worldwide have ranged from treating weight loss and arthritis to lowering high cholesterol. In fact, 80 percent of people who

times a day. Fenugreek, which has a bittersweet taste, is best sprinkled on food or sipped as an herbal tea. Steep one teaspoon of ground seed in one cup of freshly boiled water. If you don't like its taste, take one or two 580-milligram capsules of fenugreek three or four times a day for the same LDL-lowering results.

Hot Flashes

In no time flat, a hot flash can work you into a sweat. In just a matter of seconds, this abrupt sensation of sweat and heat drenches your face, neck, chest, and sometimes, your entire body.

took guggul in one study lowered their cholesterol by 24 percent. In addition, their triglycerides—another form of blood fat—dropped 23 percent.

Geraldine's next step would be to bring the information she has gathered on her next visit to her doctor. Once he has looked through it, he may surprise her with his reaction. More and more doctors are open to recommending herbal remedies now that there is so much public interest in alternative medicine. If Geraldine's doctor isn't open to her at least trying guggul, she should find out why. He may have a good reason for his point of view. If she still feels strongly about giving it a shot even after hearing her doctor out, maybe she should consider finding a doctor who is less close-minded.

Whatever Geraldine decides, she should continue to have her cholesterol levels checked every three months. And she should avoid guggul if she has an ulcer, heavy menstrual flow, or problems with acid reflux—a cause of heartburn. Guggul can aggravate these conditions.

Expert consulted
Nancy Lonsdorf, M.D.
Ayurvedic practitioner
Medical director of the Maharishi Vedic
Medical Center
Rockville, Maryland

Shivering chills follow as your body reacts to wide-open pores and soaked skin.

Of all the changes heralding menopause, most women rate these heated surges as the most notorious. Three out of every four American women experience them during the transition from monthly periods to menopause. They can occur anytime of the day or night.

No one knows exactly what provokes hot flashes, but some experts suggest that hormonal changes may irritate blood vessels and nerves, causing the blood vessels to overdilate. Others theorize that a hot flash kicks in when levels of the female hormone estrogen plummet.

Estrogen influences the hypothalamus, your brain's thermostat. When estrogen levels drop, your body's ability to regulate your temperature goes haywire. Blood surges to the surface of your skin. Your skin temperature rises a little, and your heartbeat and breathing speed up slightly. As your body desperately tries to cool itself, you perspire. Because the hot flash dissipates heat, your body's core temperature drops, making you feel cold and clammy. Total time elapsed: just two to five minutes.

Fortunately, hot flashes are physically harmless, but they can make you feel flustered and self-conscious—or leave you feeling irritable and fatigued if they strike while you sleep. The first few may take you by surprise, but eventually, you'll learn to anticipate their arrival. When a hot flash is on the way, reach for one of these herbal remedies.

Tame the flash with motherwort and more. To moderate hot flashes day or night, turn to motherwort and black cohosh. Mix two parts of motherwort tincture with one part black cohosh tincture. Take one-quarter teaspoon of this formula, mixed into a little water or a cup of tea, three times per day. Motherwort has been scientifically proven to strengthen your heart by lowering blood pressure. It also has sedative qualities to fight insomnia. Black cohosh contains estrogen-like substances that relieve the discomforts of hot flashes.

Cool down fast with chickweed. To reduce the severity and frequency of hot flashes, herbalists recommend 25 to 40 drops of chickweed tincture once or twice a day. Most women see improvement within a week or two of regular use.

THE HERBAL KITCHEN
Natural Ginger Ale

If you drink ginger ale because it gives you a sugar charge, buy it in a store. But if you need it to soothe an upset stomach, make your own! Try this all-natural recipe recommended by herbalist Kathi Keville, director of the American Herb Association and author of *Herbs for Health and Healing.*

 1 teaspoon fresh ginger (sliced thin), or ½ teaspoon powdered ginger
 1 teaspoon red raspberry leaves
 3 cups water
 1 cup carbonated water
 1 lemon slice

Place the ginger, red raspberry leaves, and plain water in a saucepan. Bring to a boil, then reduce the heat and simmer for 5 minutes. Remove from heat and steep 10 more minutes. Strain out the herbs. Add the carbonated water and lemon just before serving. Drink as much as you desire.

Indigestion

It could have been those three helpings of pecan pie last night, or the way you gulped down breakfast in the car on your way to work this morning. Maybe it was just stress. Whatever the cause, your stomach's burning, you feel gassy and bloated—and way too full.

Simply stated, you have indigestion. Here's what to do.

Ease the ache with peppermint. To calm your stomach and dispel gas, try a cup of peppermint tea. You will get best results by growing your own peppermint and using the fresh or dried leaves. But store-bought peppermint tea can also help. Use one tablespoon of whole dried leaves (two tablespoons of fresh leaves) or one tea bag per cup of hot water. Steep for 10 minutes. Sip slowly, allowing yourself—and your stomach—to relax. If indigestion is common, have a cup in the morning and one at night to prevent it.

Speed digestion with ginger. Soothe your stomach and aid digestion with a ginger tea. Use one teaspoon of grated ginger, steeped in a cup of just-boiled water. Strain and sip. Ginger contains gingerols and shogaols, chemicals that stimulate the wavelike muscle contractions (known as peristalsis) that move food from the stomach to the small intestine.

Sip an herbal aperitif. To stop indigestion before it starts, quaff this five-herb aperitif about 30 minutes before meals. Herbalists say this drink will prime your digestive system for your meal and help you more easily break down the food into nutrients.

Combine one ounce dried gentian root (ground and sifted), one-half ounce dried barberry (ground and sifted), one-half ounce dried angelica (ground and sifted), one-quarter ounce crushed dried fennel seeds, and one-quarter ounce crushed dried cardamom seeds in a glass container with a tight lid. When you're not using them, store in a cool location. Before a big meal, add one teaspoon of the herb mix to one cup of boiling water. Cover and simmer for 15 minutes. Allow the tea to cool, then strain. Have one-half cup 30 minutes before a meal. (You can refrigerate the other half-cup, covered, to use the next day.) Drink this aperitif tea warm or cold, to your taste, but don't add ice. Ice will suppress digestion and hamper these herbs from doing their job. Dried gentian root and dried angelica may be difficult to find so check with your naturo-pathic physician.

Finish with fennel. At the close of a big meal, ward off indigestion by chewing a teaspoon of fennel. The naturally bitter taste gets your digestive juices flowing. It's a traditional choice in India and is often offered after meals at Indian restaurants in the United States.

Infertility

Long before the emergence of fertility drugs, ovulation test kits, sperm analysis, and infertility clinics, women relied on plant remedies in the hope of reversing infertility and finally bearing children.

Many fertility herbs used today come to us from ancient Chinese and Native American herbal medicine traditions. Experts in alternative medicine recommend matching good nutrition, exercise, and stress reduction with herbs to enhance fertility so that your body is in prime condition to conceive—and hold on to—the fragile beginnings of life.

If you want to reverse infertility, you'll have to figure out what's causing it. Rule out the most obvious possibilities first: You're fertile but your husband is not, you're underweight (fat levels below one-quarter of your total body weight often stop ovulation), you're too stressed, or you haven't timed intercourse to coincide with your most fertile time of the month.

Lots of physical conditions can cause infertility. Possibilities include endometriosis, uterine fibroids, lack of ovulation, or Fallopian tubes scarred by sexually transmitted diseases, such as chlamydia and gonorrhea. Age is also a factor. Fertility drops after age 35, and more sharply after age 40.

Work with your doctor to determine what's going on in your particular case. Some women need surgery or drug treatments to improve their fertility. For other women, herbal remedies can help balance hormone levels and restore overall vitality—which may be sufficient to help you conceive. Here's how.

Sip a six-herb formula. To enhance fertility, drink two cups of this fertility tea daily: In a pot, combine one teaspoon each dried dong quai (also known as dang gui), Siberian ginseng, and chasteberry (also known as vitex) with one teaspoon each dried motherwort leaves, cramp bark, and wild yam in one quart of water. Simmer for 5 minutes. Turn off the heat and steep for 20 minutes. Strain out the herbs before drinking.

Dong quai and cramp bark relax the uterus and help regulate menstrual irregularities. Siberian ginseng fights stress. Chasteberry helps balance hormones. Motherwort is used for a variety of female conditions, and wild yam is reputed to have estrogenic effects.

Over 40? Start with dandelion. If you're over 40 and want to have a baby, herbalists often recommend you start by revitalizing your body by taking bitters like dandelion root before meals. Try 5 to 10 drops of dandelion root tincture right before you eat. Add bitter "gourmet" greens, such as dandelion leaves and arugula, to your salads, too. Since your body slows down the production of enzymes as you age, an older prospective mom may need to boost her body's ability to absorb nutrients before trying fertility-enhancing herbs. Research shows dandelion contains bitter compounds that stimulate the secretion of bile, which aids in digestion.

GARLIC
Good for: bacterial and fungal infections, digestive ailments, and high blood pressure

WOMEN ASK WHY

If hops is the main ingredient in beer and an herb used to cure insomnia, why does drinking beer perk me up instead of put me to sleep?

While drinking a few beers may give you a little jump start, that's not hops working—that's alcohol. Within moments of drinking beer, alcohol reaches your brain, where it stimulates your system and produces feelings of euphoria. That's why you get a quick pick-me-up.

Give the beer time, of course, and it may just put you to sleep. Although alcohol stimulates you at first, it soon starts acting as a depressant. As the euphoria ebbs, a sedating effect takes its place, producing calmness and tranquillity. Depending on how much you drink, alcohol will ultimately induce a hypnotic state and sleep. In fact, alcohol is considered a tranquilizer and a member of the sedative-hypnotic drug family.

By contrast, if you try some hops tea or tincture before turning in for the night, or even if you make a hops pillow for yourself, you'll feel the sedative effects that cure insomnia. The herb also relieves tension, anxiety, pain, restlessness, and agitation.

Expert consulted
Mindy Green
A founding and professional member
*   of the American Herbalists Guild*
Coauthor of Aromatherapy: A Complete
*   Guide to the Healing Art*
Director of the Herb Research Foundation
Boulder, Colorado

Insomnia

Coast to coast, some 20 to 50 million Americans regularly miss out on a good night's rest. Some take a long time to doze off. Others wake up from sleep repeatedly during the night. Still others fall into dreamland quickly, only to wake at 2:00 A.M., when they find themselves unable to fall back to sleep.

Sleepless nights usually turn into sleepy days. Women, more than men, need between 8 and 8½ hours of sleep each night. Losing even an hour or so each night can rob you of your normal get-up-and-go. You may lack energy, drive, and concentration, or find that you become irritated more easily.

Lifestyle adjustments such as avoiding coffee at night and exercising a few times a week can help fight insomnia. So can meditation and progressive relaxation techniques. Natural healers also suggest these good-night herbs for a good night's sleep.

Cap the night with lemon balm. For a safe sedative that also soothes your stomach, herbalists suggest a cup of lemon balm tea at bedtime. Use one to three teaspoons of the dried herb per cup of just-boiled water. Cover, steep for 10 minutes, and strain. Chemicals in the plant, called terpenes, help provide a sedative action.

Find slumber with valerian. If you're looking for an herbal alternative to tranquilizers, select valerian. The herb's active ingredient includes a group of compounds called valepotriates. Research shows that these compounds attach to the same brain receptors as tranquilizers. Valerian is not one of the best-tasting or smelling herbs, so herbalists recommend you take one or two 400-milligram capsules (rather than tea or tincture) about 30 minutes before bed for best results.

Begin the morning with a relaxing herb. Don't wait until bedtime to take herbs that soothe the nervous system and promote restful sleep. By keeping calm all day, you'll find it much easier to slip into dreamland after dark. Choose either passionflower, skullcap, or St. John's wort. Use one tablespoon of dried herb per cup of just-boiled water. Steep for an hour, strain, and sip.

GINGER
Good for: motion sickness, nausea, and menstrual cramps

Jet Lag

Whether you're traveling for business or pleasure, jet lag can leave you feeling foggy-headed and physically sapped.

When you fly across several time zones, it takes time for your internal body clock to adjust to the new local day/night cycle. Until it resets itself, you may feel irritable and experience headaches, fatigue, an upset stomach, or insomnia. Traveling from east to west, say from New York to Honolulu, is easier on your internal clock than journeying west to east. That's because you're pushing your body clock backward instead of forward. Sleep disorder specialists say that it's easier to stay up later—and wake up later—than to try to sleep earlier and get up earlier.

On its own, your body needs about one day of adjustment for every time zone you cross. But if you're taking a short vacation, you might not be fully adjusted until it's time to board the plane home. You can gently encourage your internal

clock to reset more quickly and help yourself adjust more comfortably to your new surroundings with these herbal travel helpers.

Adapt with ginseng. Aid your adjustment to new surroundings in a different time zone by taking 250 milligrams of Siberian ginseng in capsule form twice daily. Start taking Siberian ginseng four days before a long flight, then take it during the flight and for four days after you arrive at your destination. This herb will help overcome the stress of adapting to a new time zone.

Tuck fragrant herbs in your pillow. For peaceful sleep upon arrival, dab a drop each of the essential oils ylang-ylang, lavender, and frankincense on a tissue, according to herbal experts. Tuck the tissue under your pillow and get some well-deserved zzzs. Ylang-ylang wards off depression and nervous tension; lavender eases insomnia; and frankincense is believed to soothe the spirit. If traveling disrupts your menstrual cycle or makes PMS worse, add a drop of rose geranium to the formula. This herb helps normalize hormones.

Arrive alert with essential oils. If you need to be sharp and alert as soon as you step off of the plane, aromatherapy experts suggest you pack these energizing essential oils: rosemary, basil, eucalyptus, and peppermint. Dab a drop of each on a tissue or handkerchief. Breathe in every time your eyelids start to close. Rosemary stimulates your nervous system; basil overcomes mental fatigue; eucalyptus is an energy booster; and peppermint counters mental fogginess.

Pack herbal tea bags. In addition to your suitcases, don't forget to pack chamomile tea bags. Dunk the tea bags in cool water and place them on the skin just below your eyes to combat fatigue-induced puffiness. Drink a cup of chamomile tea once you arrive to help you relax after a long and stressful trip.

Laryngitis

The mouth opens, the lips and tongue form words, but the voice . . . where's the voice? That rasping croak that comes out instead really *could* be from a frog who sets up housekeeping in throats. Don't panic. It's only laryngitis.

Similar to a sore throat, laryngitis dries out the mucous membranes that surround the larynx, or the voice box. When this membrane can't moisten or filter air properly, your speaking voice—created by air passing over your vocal cords—becomes whispery or totally disappears. A cold or flu, excessive shouting, or even singing can cause voice loss.

Fortunately, herbal healers say you can regain your voice with herbs.

Say it with herbal steam. When a virus or excessive talking robs you of your voice, heal your larynx and vocal cords naturally with an essential-oil steam. Bring three cups of water to a simmer and turn off the heat. Add one-quarter teaspoon of eucalyptus or peppermint essential oil. Place the pot in front of you. Position your face over the pot at a distance so that the steam doesn't burn your face and drape a towel over the back of your head to form a mini-sauna. Breathe in the steam for 10 to 15 minutes, coming out for fresh air as needed.

Do this at least three times a day. Eucalyptus contains a chemical called cineole that researchers believe may relieve sore throat inflammation and fight infection. Peppermint contains

MAKING AN HERBAL SLEEP PILLOW

Since the dawn of time, people have relied on herb-filled pillows to lull them to sleep.

Two thousand years ago, people were using chamomile to soothe both the physical and mental irritations that kept them up at night. During the Middle Ages, lavender remedied stress, hysteria, and headaches. In the eighteenth century, physicians for mad King George III put hops in his pillow to help him to rest.

Tucked away inside a small sack, these herbs, which are believed to heal the nervous system, chased away restlessness and insomnia, says herbalist Rosemary Gladstar, director of the Sage Mountain Herbal Education Center in East Barre, Vermont, and author of *Herbal Healing for Women*.

You can make your own herbal pillow and give yourself the gift of a peaceful night's rest. There are two types: sleep pillows and dream pillows, Gladstar says. A sleep pillow specifically induces sleep. A dream pillow also brings on slumber, but it stimulates your dreams as well.

To make a dream pillow, simply add mugwort, an herb that herbalists believe really gets you dreaming.

To make a sleep pillow, fold a piece of eight-inch by eight-inch fabric in half. Soft fabrics such as cotton, flannel, or velvet are best. If you like, embroider or decorate it. Sew two of the sides together, leaving one side open for stuffing. Make sure the fabric is inside out when you sew it.

In a bowl, mix together the following dried herbs: one part lavender, one part hops, one part chamomile, and one part rose. (Rarely, hops can cause a skin rash, so handle fresh or dried hops carefully.) If you want your sleep pillow to act also as a dream pillow, add four parts mugwort. Turn the pillow right side out, and stuff the mixture into it. Six to eight ounces of the herb mixture should be enough to fill the pillow. Sew closed the remaining open side.

Place the herbal pillow beside your head or inside your regular pillow at night. Fluff it before you go to sleep to release the odors. The pillow will last for several years, but if you like, you can renew the herbs every year.

substances believed to kill many kinds of microorganisms.

Lose laryngitis with a spicy juice. For laryngitis induced by a cold, herbalists recommend this mixture of lemons, honey, and ground red pepper. Squeeze the juice from one to two fresh lemons, then mix the juice with a tablespoon of honey and a pinch of ground red pepper. Take a small sip of the mixture every few hours throughout the day. Ground red pepper (also known as cayenne pepper) thins phlegm and eases its passage from the lungs, thus helping to prevent and treat colds.

Low Immunity

Do cold and flu germs seem to make a beeline directly to you? When others fend off the sniffles easily, are you bedridden for days? Chances are your immune system could use some recharging.

The immune system is a complex network of organs, glands, and special cells that works in harmony to protect your body against infection and disease. It aggressively seeks and destroys viruses, bacteria, and other invaders. Most of the time, the immune system works perfectly well on its own. But if you're not well-nourished, well-rested, and prepared for daily stress, your immune system won't be strong enough to continuously fend off harmful intruders. As a consequence, you get sick often.

Bolster your immune system by eating right (five to seven servings of fruits and vegetables daily, as part of an

WOMAN TO WOMAN

On-the-Go Sportswriter Always Packs Her Echinacea

Marcia Smith, a Philadelphia Inquirer sportswriter, often found herself working long hours for weeks at a stretch, traveling to different cities, and confronting different climates. The stress of all that travel, on top of pressure to produce great writing and meet deadlines, began to take a toll on her immune system. Cold viruses zeroed in on her. She had become easy prey. This is the story of how she fought back.

In my job, I can't afford to miss a day sick in bed with a cold. But unfortunately, I'm prone to catching colds because I'm constantly in and out of airports, airplanes, hotels, stadiums, and locker rooms—all places where people are constantly shedding germs. It doesn't help that I don't have regular eating or sleeping habits.

About a year ago, both my mom, who's a clinical chemist, and a good friend of mine, who's a medical school student, suggested I start taking echinacea as soon as I feel a cold coming on. Like me, both of them are in high-energy professions, and they rarely get sick. They explained that echinacea strengthens the immune system and may help me fight off a cold a lot better than over-the-counter medications. So I bought a bottle of caplets from a local health food store.

I really needed the caplets during the height of the cold and flu season recently. After working a full Friday reporting on the Philadelphia Eagles, I drove five hours to Hartford, Connecticut, to cover the University of Connecticut men's basketball team's pre-season midnight practice. I arrived in Hartford at 9:00 P.M., tired, hungry, and feeling a cold coming on. So I made sure I took echinacea with the pasta dinner room service brought to me. Then, I went to the arena to cover the team's first practice. The next day, I took more echinacea with my meals. I believe it helped me hold off a cold until I got the time to rest and heal on my own.

I don't take echinacea all the time—only at the first signs of a cold or cough. I know this isn't the way it really works, but I feel as if this herb puts armor on my white blood cells. Since I've started taking echinacea, I haven't had a cold or needed to take a sick day off from work.

eating plan that also emphasizes whole grains and low-fat protein sources), doing regular exercise (such as walking 30 minutes at least five days a week), getting sufficient rest (eight hours each night), and using stress management. Then add these herbal boosters.

Fortify with ginseng. Give your immune system a helping hand, especially during cold and flu season, with Siberian ginseng or panax ginseng (sometimes called Asian or Korean ginseng). Two or three times a day, take 40 to 60 drops of Siberian ginseng tincture mixed into a little water. Or try taking 20 to 40 drops of panax ginseng (often simply called ginseng on product labels) in water two or three times a day.

Studies show that Russian factory workers who used Siberian ginseng during cold and flu season took fewer sick days. Siberian ginseng contains substances that fuel the adrenal glands and help them to withstand emotional and physical stresses. It also contains compounds that fight viruses. Panax ginseng contains another group of compounds believed to stimulate immunity.

Enlist the immune-system boosters. Help bolster your resistance to illness with the immune-strengthening powers of echinacea and other fortifying herbs. Combine one-half teaspoon each of tinctures of echinacea root, pau d'arco bark, Siberian ginseng root, licorice root, astragalus root, and bupleurum root.

Take this twice a day for a few weeks to fortify your immune system.

Arm germ-fighting cells with garlic. Fresh garlic cloves can be a faithful friend to an overworked immune system. Eat two cloves of fresh garlic every day. Garlic enhances your immune system by recharging your natural killer cells, white blood cells that seek and destroy disease-causing invaders. Mask the garlic odor by chewing on some parsley afterward.

Low Sexual Desire

Imagine desiring him so much that your breasts tingle and your heart flutters. Imagine feeling this passion—tonight. You can capture that "swept away" feeling, herbalists say, with the help of herbal potions, oils, and teas.

Inhale a sensual aroma. To set the mood for passion, scent your bedroom (or any room) with a few potent drops of sandalwood, rose, or amber essential oil. Just add a few drops of essential oil to a cup of warm water (the heat will release the aroma) or place five drops of essential oil and one-half cup of water in an atomizer, then shake and spray into the air. Sandalwood is a traditional aphrodisiac that makes you feel very centered in your body. Rose and amber have long had reputations for evoking sensuality.

Sip this love-enhancing tea. Boost blood circulation to the pelvic area with spicy, passion-producing tea. Simmer the following herbs in two cups of water for 20 minutes: one tablespoon of grated gingerroot, 7 to 10 clove buds, two to three cinnamon sticks, four to five peppercorns, and 7 to 10 cardamom pods. Strain and add small amounts of milk and honey to taste. Top it with one-quarter teaspoon of vanilla, a member of the orchid family known for being an aphrodisiac. Then enjoy this tea with your partner in a warm bath surrounded by beautiful candles. See where it leads. . . .

Memory Problems and Poor Concentration

Ever find yourself rereading the same paragraph in a gripping mystery novel several times and still not recalling what it said? Do you tend to forget where you placed your car keys or find yourself in a supermarket aisle, unable to remember what you needed to buy? Ever blank on a friend's name in the middle of an introduction?

Don't worry. Minor memory lapses and simple concentration slipups happen to everyone—they don't mean you're losing your memory. Forgetfulness and fuzzy thinking are often linked to stress, fatigue, and outright exhaustion. Some women also complain of temporary memory loss during menopause, especially if they experience night sweats and are unable to get enough sleep.

Emotionally charged events—childbirth, divorce, job loss, or the death of a loved one—can impair anyone's memory at any age. Stress causes the adrenal glands to release cortisol, a hormone that enables you to get through sudden emergencies. But over time, constant stress gradually kills or injures billions of brain cells, interfering with your ability to think and concentrate.

Once you've accounted for (and corrected) external factors that may be blunting your thinking, sharpen your memory and concentration further with these herbal helpers.

Give your brain a healthy workout with ginkgo. Improve blood flow to the brain and enhance your brain's ability to use oxygen by taking 120 to 240 milligrams of ginkgo a day, di-

GINSENG
Good for: stress, fatigue, and memory loss as well as protecting the liver

At the National College of Naturopathic Medicine in Portland, Oregon, students sometimes show up for class wearing wreaths of rosemary around their necks, especially when they're about to take a big test.

Is this some sort of herbal crib sheet? Or just a lucky charm, like a four-leaf clover or rabbit's foot? Not quite. According to Sharleen Andrews-Miller, a faculty member at the college, the scent of any of several common botanicals might be just the boost their brains need to keep their memories sharp. Those students know what they're doing!

Of course, most of us would prefer not to wear our herbs like a necklace, so something like a basil memory jar might be a better choice. Like rosemary, basil is thought to be a great brain booster. And kept in a jar, it will last longer, be easier to transport, and draw far less attention.

To make your own basil memory jar, stuff three or four cotton balls into a one-ounce glass jar with a lid. Using a dropper, put three to five drops of basil essential oil into the jar, spreading the drops among the cotton balls. Screw the lid tightly onto the jar. When you need a memory or an alertness boost, open the jar and sniff the scent. Be sure to close the lid tightly, or the essential oil will dry out. Replace when the smell becomes faint.

vided into two doses. Dozens of studies in Germany and France have substantiated that ginkgo is an excellent herb for improving memory, especially for seniors. Make sure to select ginkgo tablets that are standardized to contain 24 percent ginkgo flavone glycosides and 6 percent terpene lactones—two of ginkgo's most important active ingredients.

Smell rosemary for remembrance. For minor concentration lapses and forgetfulness, sniff the scent of rosemary essential oil. Just apply one to three drops to a tissue, tuck it in your pocket or purse, and inhale as needed. This herb's ability to improve memory and concentra-

tion dates back centuries. In Shakespeare's *Hamlet*, the mad Ophelia declares, "There's rosemary, that's for remembrance."

Try a concentration-boosting formula. When you need to concentrate extra-hard for an important meeting or exam, this formula will improve your ability to focus. Combine one teaspoon each of the tinctures of ginkgo and Siberian ginseng with one-half teaspoon each of tinctures of panax ginseng (also called Asian ginseng) and gotu kola. Take half a dropperful a few times a day and have an extra dose an hour before the big event.

Clinical studies show that these four herbs enhance mental abilities, including concentration, aptitude, alertness, and even intelligence.

Menopause

Today, as baby boomers move into midlife by the millions, menopause is recognized as a normal stage in life and not a disease. Many regard menopause as puberty in reverse, a time when you finally no longer need to worry about menstrual periods or birth control.

Strictly speaking, menopause means that you haven't had a menstrual period for a year, but well before that happens, you'll experience many changes. Since puberty, your body has amply produced the female hormones estrogen and progesterone. But by age 50, smaller and smaller amounts of these hormones are secreted, so eventually menstruation ceases.

As hormone production dwindles, you may experience hot flashes, insomnia, irregular bleeding, mood swings, vaginal dryness, and other changes. Every woman experiences a unique combination of physical and emotional changes during this transition time.

Conventional medicine treats menopause as a deficiency disease of estrogen. Although doctors often prescribe hormone-replacement therapy (HRT), replacement hormones can't fully mimic your body's natural cycle. And some women stop taking HRT after experiencing the side effects, which can include menstrual-like bleeding, bloating, irritability, cramps, headaches, and depression.

Natural alternatives can help minimize menopausal symptoms. Consuming 30 to 50 milligrams of isoflavones, found in soy foods such as tofu or soy milk or tempeh, each day seems to blunt bothersome hot flashes and vaginal dryness. Isoflavones are weak, plant-derived forms of estrogen. Engaging in regular aerobic activity helps combat weight gain, heart disease, and osteoporosis, conditions for which a woman's risk increases following menopause. Experts recommend that you exercise for at least 30 minutes, two to three times a week (walking is ideal).

Besides dietary and lifestyle changes, certain herbs can protect your health as you go through menopause.

Try a combination blend. If you experience several change-of-life symptoms, look for multi-herb products formulated specifically for menopause. These usually contain some combination of the following

REAL-LIFE SCENARIO
On-Again, Off-Again Menopause

Like many of her friends, Elizabeth had problems when she started to go through menopause. Her periods came when least expected—if at all. They alternated between being very light and so heavy that she had to take a change of clothes to work. Finally, they stopped altogether, but the hot flashes and night sweats continued. Plus, her mood started to change—she became frequently irritable and headachy. She decided to seek a natural remedy for her problems and eventually found great relief from using black cohosh. Everything seemed settled. But this morning, she got her period again. Could this herb be the reason?

The rise and fall of certain hormones in our bodies—primarily estrogen—dictates our monthly cycles. When levels of estrogen decline, so does the frequency of our periods. Black cohosh produces substances that can act like estrogen, so the body gets fooled. In Elizabeth's case, the higher levels of "estrogen" brought on by the herb caused her body to start menstruating again.

Although it probably annoys her, the return of menstruation actually acts to her advantage. As long as she menstruates, she knows her body still has enough estrogen to protect her from developing heart disease and osteoporosis. The black cohosh alone would not cause her to menstruate if her own hormones were at the very low levels associated with post-menopause.

Of course, if Elizabeth experienced premenstrual symptoms in the past, they may also start up again. Fortunately, they aren't likely to be as severe. That's because the plant form of estrogen isn't nearly as strong as the hormone your body produces.

All in all, it looks as if black cohosh is doing exactly what it's supposed to for Elizabeth. It's a therapy she would do well to continue.

Expert consulted
Lorilee Schoenbeck, N.D.
Naturopathic physician
Champlain Center for Natural Medicine
Shelburne, Vermont

WOMAN TO WOMAN

An Herbal Blend Relieves Her of Her Menstrual Woes

After the birth of her son, Susan Fisher, a 37-year-old caterer and computer student from Pittstown, New Jersey, began to experience extremely bad cramps and heavy blood flow during her monthly periods. Then she started taking a botanical blend prepared by an herbalist, and things began to change. This is her story.

For as long as I can remember, I always had bad cramps and heavy bleeding during my monthly periods. I thought that was just the way my body was. But then, after the birth of my son, Ryan (who is now nine), the bleeding and cramping got worse. Blood clots were coming out like silver dollars. I'd insert a tampon and five minutes later, I needed to replace it. I was scared.

I went to a gynecologist who gave me a prescription to stop the bleeding. But I learned there were many funky side effects possible. For example, my periods could become terribly irregular, and when they did come, the bleeding might last for 10 days. This turned me off. I wanted to find something more natural, so I decided not to fill that prescription.

A friend of mine suggested that I see a local herbalist named Kerry Adams. After talking with me in detail, Kerry said she felt I was getting such wicked periods because my liver was congested. So she prepared a tincture. The one-ounce bottle contained a mixture of dandelion root, turmeric, chasteberry, Oregon grape root, and wild yam extracts. I just had to shake it, squeeze some into a little water or juice, and drink it a few times every day. By my second period, my belly no longer felt crampy, and I was replacing tampons every hour instead of every five minutes.

Everything feels back in check now. Once in a long while, I have a little cramping, but nothing so bad that it makes me want to lie in bed for two days like I did before. I have much more energy to spend on my son, who is very bright and a joy to be around.

Herbs are wonderful. I know they have helped my life. But I also realize that herbs are just like medicines, so I always check with Kerry before taking any new herb.

strengthening and hormone-balancing herbs: chasteberry, black cohosh, dong quai, panax ginseng (also called Asian or Korean ginseng), and licorice root. These herbs balance and complement each other, which enhances their effectiveness and reduces side effects. For the most consistent results, look for blends that contain standardized extracts.

Stop mood swings with skullcap. Counter uncontrollable crying, angry outbursts, or other mood swings associated with menopause by taking skullcap twice a day. Use four to eight drops of skullcap tincture every morning and evening when you feel fried, stressed-out, wired, or just wound up. Skullcap strengthens the nerves, eases sensitivity, and helps promote deep, sound sleep.

Cool hot flashes with black cohosh. Research shows that black cohosh, an herb that was used traditionally by Native Americans, is as effective as estrogen for the relief of hot flashes. To find the best dosage, herbalists suggest starting with 10 drops of black cohosh tincture twice a day and increasing the dose by 5 drops every other day until you're satisfied with the results. You may take it, as needed, for two weeks out of every month.

Menstrual Cramps and Bloating

Womanhood is a wonderful thing. But one part of it, those body-bending cramps we get during the first hours or days of our periods, is not.

Cramps are the result of a release of hormones called prostaglandins that cause uterine blood vessels to tighten, reducing blood flow. This makes the uterine muscle flex in what you feel as a painful cramp. As for bloating, blame it on a drop in the female hormone progesterone in the 7 to 10 days before your menstrual cycle. Depletion of progesterone causes salt and water retention throughout your body.

Women herbalists offer these botanical remedies that regulate hormones so that cramping and bloating become less severe.

Stop cramps quickly with cramp bark and valerian. If you're suffering from intense cramps and need relief right now, herbalists suggest blending three teaspoons of cramp bark tincture and five teaspoons of valerian tincture. Then take between 40 drops and one teaspoon of this blend in small amounts of warm water up to three times a day if necessary. Cramp bark relaxes muscles and soothes painful spasms. Valerian contains compounds that relieve muscle spasms and curb anxiety.

Ease pain with black haw. If menstrual cramps leave you doubled over in pain, herbal experts advocate taking black haw before pain peaks. This herb contains an aspirin-like compound that lessens the pain. Make a tea by adding two teaspoons of dried black haw per cup of water. Boil 10 minutes, cool, strain, and drink up to three cups a day. Women practitioners say it's best to start taking this tea a few days before you expect your period—don't wait until the pain becomes overwhelming.

Dodge discomfort with tea. Some women can lessen or even prevent menstrual cramps by drinking a hormone-balancing blend. To make the tea, combine one-quarter part dried chasteberry with one part each of dried wild yam, ginger, and yellow dock. Add two parts each dried dandelion root, burdock, licorice, and sassafras. Brew the tea by adding six tablespoons of the blend to a quart of cold water in a pot.

Simmer slowly for 20 minutes, then strain. Drink three to four cups daily for three weeks during each menstrual cycle, then stop while you menstruate. Long-term use of sassafras is not recommended; do not take more than the recommended dose.

These herbs help keep the liver healthy, an organ that is key to a woman's reproductive health. They promote bile flow so the liver can better process hormones. This blend also improves circulation, aids digestion, and fights uterine pain and cramping.

Halt bloating with dandelion. Dandelion leaves, a potent diuretic, effectively reduce uncomfortable bloating and swelling before and during menstruation. This herb also helps cleanse and rejuvenate the liver and promotes healthy digestion. Check with your naturopathic physician for availability and dosage.

GOLDENSEAL
Good for: sinus infections, colds and flu, laryngitis, sore throats, earaches, gastritis, and colitis

Menstrual Flow, Heavy

Slight changes in your monthly menstrual flow are normal and may be brought on by lifestyle changes—such as starting a new job, beginning a new exercise routine, or moving into a new home. Age could also be a factor. Until around age 35, your uterus keeps growing, so there's more uterine lining to shed during menstruation. But as you approach menopause in your forties and fifties, monthly periods can become unpredictable. Heavy blood flow can drain your energy, lower your blood pressure, and intensify menstrual cramps.

Women doctors urge you to pay attention to your monthly cycle so you know what's normal for you. Jot down when your period starts and ends, and record your blood flow as heavy, medium, or light. It's especially important to see your doctor if heavy bleeding makes you feel light-headed, if you start passing blood clots, or if the heavy flow soaks through a pad or tampon every hour for 12 to 24 hours. Heavy bleeding that comes on suddenly may signal a miscarriage. Extra blood loss may also lead to anemia, an iron deficiency condition that makes you feel weak and weary.

After your physician rules out possible underlying medical causes for your heavy bleeding, herbalists recommend a two-prong strategy. Select some herbs to slow and regulate the flow and others to help correct hormone imbalances that can cause heavy bleeding.

Seek relief from yarrow and the gang. Stop an episode of excessive menstrual bleeding with the astringent herbs shepherd's purse, yarrow, geranium root, and lady's-mantle. Herbalists recommend a formula that combines two parts shepherd's purse tincture with one part each of the tinctures of yarrow, geranium, and lady's-mantle. Take one-half to one teaspoon three or four times a day when menstrual flow is heavy.

Come to the aid of your liver. You can help correct hormone imbalances by feeding your liver, which processes certain hormones. Burdock, dandelion, fennel, and milk thistle are traditionally used for liver support. Milk thistle, the subject of more than 300 studies, contains silymarin, a substance that helps protect liver cells from toxic chemicals and at the same time stimulates the growth of new liver cells.

Create your own hormone-balancing, liver-friendly formula by using one or two of the following dried herbs: dandelion, milk thistle, burdock, or fennel. Brew a tea using one tea-spoon of herb or herb mix per cup of boiling water, steep 15 to 20 minutes, and strain. Have two to three cups a day. If a cup of tea isn't your cup of tea, you can take one 200-milligram milk thistle capsule two or three times a day. Or you can combine equal parts of the tinctures of your chosen liver herbs and have one teaspoon of the mix three times a day. Take liver-friendly herbs for several months.

LAVENDER
Good for: headaches, muscle spasms and cramps, depression, and digestive upsets

Menstrual Period Irregularity

A woman's menstrual cycle doesn't always run on schedule. Illness, stress, travel, and aging can cause month-to-month fluctuations. For example, women in their twenties tend to have longer cycles, while women over 35 usually have shorter cycles because of hormonal changes.

At the start of a normal menstrual cycle, hormones prompt one or more eggs in the ovary to mature. By midcycle, one egg bursts from its follicle and sails down the Fallopian tube into the uterus. If it is fertilized during the journey, a pregnancy may begin. If not, menstruation starts. While some say this sequence of events normally occurs over 28 days, medical experts say the reality is that normal menstrual cycles for women can range in length from 21 to 38 days.

Be sure to discuss your menstrual cycle with your gynecologist during your yearly visit just to be certain everything is normal. If your cycle is truly irregular—dramatically shorter one month, longer the next—then these herbal remedies can help restore regularity.

Feed your reproductive system with a tonic tea. Take steps to regulate your cycle by first nourishing your reproductive system with a female tonic tea. This refreshing vitamin- and mineral-rich tea contains raspberry leaf, nettle, peppermint, and other herbs.

Make this tea by mixing two parts each dried raspberry leaf, nettle, peppermint leaf, and lemongrass (for flavor), with one part each dried strawberry leaf and lady's-mantle. Add a pinch of stevia to sweeten the mixture, if desired. Brew the tea by adding six tablespoons of the mix to a quart of cold water in a saucepan. Bring to a low boil. Remove from the heat and steep for 20 minutes. Strain the herbs and drink three to four cups a day.

Get back on track with chasteberry. If hormonal imbalances turn the anticipated arrival date of your next monthly period into a guessing game, try restoring your schedule with chasteberry. This herb is commonly prescribed in Europe to regulate menstrual cycles.

Chasteberry, sometimes called vitex, seems to work through the pituitary gland, your body's master gland, to help reestablish hormonal balance.

Take a dropperful of chasteberry tincture two or three times a day in a small glass of warm water for six to eight weeks. Stop this daily routine during menstruation and resume when bleeding has stopped. Your menstrual cycle should become more regular within two to four months.

Find sweet harmony with licorice root. For a sweet-tasting tea with a well-rounded hormone-balancing effect, blend licorice root with chasteberry. Some herbalists say licorice root regulates and normalizes hormone production. To make a tea blend, use one-half teaspoon each

of dried chasteberry and licorice root. Simmer lightly for 15 minutes in one cup of water. Strain; drink three cups a day for two to four menstrual cycles.

Midafternoon Slump

In offices and homes across the country—and the world—a whole lot of yawning, stretching, and fighting off of sleep (or giving in to it) begins at about 2:00 P.M. Welcome to midafternoon, a natural siesta time for your body and mind.

Between 1:00 and 5:00 P.M., your brain and body function on minimum power. Mental focus fades. Blood sugar levels drop. Nerves fray. It's a natural, human rhythm: Within each 24-hour cycle, your body has two natural sleep periods—a long one at night and a short one at midafternoon. Small wonder, then, that some societies simply shut down for a few hours of midafternoon repose each day. But while a brief afternoon snooze will often revive you, who has time?

These herbs may help restore your mental focus, balance your blood sugar levels, and soothe frazzled nerves.

Inhale a high-energy scent. For a natural midafternoon pick-me-up, inhale the scent of rosemary, orange peel, or peppermint essential oil. Shake one or two drops of your chosen scent onto a hankie. Hold it close to your nose and inhale. You can also use a diffuser, a pump that blows the essential oil's scent into the air. Put the diffuser at your desk in your office or in your living room at home and turn it on when you feel in need of a pick-me-up.

Revive your energy with a mint-family tea. If you're sluggish by midafternoon, reach for a cup of mint tea, not coffee. Peppermint, spearmint, and lemon balm, all members of the mint family, are known for their ability to restore your energy. Use one teaspoon of your chosen dried herb per cup of boiling water. Steep for 5 to 15 minutes, covered. Lemon balm is a perfect choice for times when you feel tired yet stressed, herbalists say. If you find yourself tired every afternoon, make a thermos of your tea in advance and sip it slowly throughout the day.

Level blood sugar with dandelion. To balance blood sugar levels—and avoid sudden energy slumps—drink a cup of dandelion root tea. Boil one heaping teaspoon of dried dandelion root in 1½ cups of water for 15 to 20 minutes.

Migraines

If most ordinary headaches feel like a jeweler's hammer tapping on your temples, then a migraine feels like a sledgehammer pounding on your cranium.

Migraines, the most painful and debilitating of headaches, may stick around for several hours or even several days, causing nausea, vomiting, loss of appetite, and extreme sensitivity to light and sound—in addition to intense head pain. Like hurricanes, these intense headaches often give warnings of their approach. About 30 minutes before a migraine kicks in, your vision may blur, or you'll see bright spots. Your thinking may become jumbled. You may also feel numbness or tingling along one side of your body.

Unlike tension headaches, which are caused by muscle contractions, migraines are caused by the contraction of veins. Women experience them most often during their periods; doctors attribute this to changing levels of the hormone estrogen. If your headache problem has never been diagnosed by your doctor, it's best to have yourself checked. Headaches are sometimes symptoms of other problems.

Herbal remedies can help prevent migraines or reduce their frequency, say herbalists. Here's how.

Fight back with feverfew. If you're prone to migraines, you can get relief with a daily dose of feverfew. Take one-half teaspoon of feverfew tincture or 500 milligrams in capsule form once a day. Research demonstrates that even small amounts of feverfew can prevent the pain of these awful headaches.

Eat ginger daily. Keep blood vessels in good shape with this common kitchen spice. Ginger inhibits a substance that prevents your blood vessels from dilating. There are many ways to fit ginger into your daily eating plan, herbalists say. You can grate fresh ginger into juice, munch on Japanese pickled ginger (available at health food stores), use fresh or powdered ginger while cooking, or snack on crystallized ginger candy.

Motion Sickness

Seasickness can ruin a day of sailing faster than the doldrums.

Seasickness is just one form of motion sickness. Planes, trains, buses, and automobiles can bring on the same kind of queasiness. Motion sickness strikes when your brain receives conflicting messages about what's happening to your body. Suppose you're on a vacation flight to Orlando when the plane suddenly encounters severe turbulence. Your eyes signal to your brain that it *looks* as if you're sitting still. But your inner ear (which plays a role in balance) senses movement and tells your brain that you're moving forward—fast. The resulting

LEMON BALM
Good for: relieving depression, insomnia, nervousness, tension headaches, and digestive problems related to stress

confusion can bring on that I'd-rather-be-dead feeling of nausea, plus vomiting, cold sweats, and headaches.

If you're prone to this uncomfortable and inconvenient condition, you don't have to decline travel invitations in order to avoid nausea. With the right herbs, you can enjoy the motion without the sickness.

Take along ginger. This spicy root is the top choice of herbalists for soothing upset stomachs and preventing motion sickness. Herbalists suggest you take two 500-milligram capsules of ginger about 30 minutes before departure and then one to two more capsules if symptoms begin to occur, about every four hours. Studies show ginger works better than dimenhydrinate, the active ingredient in over-the-counter motion sickness medications such as Dramamine. Researchers think that ginger works by decreasing stomach movements caused by motion sickness or by shutting down impulses to the brain that deliver messages about equilibrium.

Select peppermint. If ginger is not available, the next best motion sickness fighter is peppermint. Although not as effective as ginger, peppermint can also soothe your nausea. About an hour before your trip, make a peppermint tea by pouring just-boiled water over a tablespoon of fresh peppermint in a cup. Cover it to keep the volatile oils from escaping and let it stand for five minutes. Strain and drink.

Be sure to bring along premade peppermint tea in your travel mug for a nausea-free trip.

Muscle Cramps

In 1996, Amy Van Dyken surprised the world by winning four gold medals in swimming events during the summer Olympic Games in Atlanta. She had overcome asthma and illness to become one of the greatest woman athletes in the history of the Olympics. But in her very first event, a 100-meter freestyle race, she finished only fourth. And when this superb athlete, at the peak of her conditioning, pulled herself out of the water, she collapsed to the deck of the pool, writhing in pain from a body-length muscle cramp.

Muscle cramps are sudden, sharp, painful contractions of the muscle fibers. In healthy women, cramping often results from overexertion and dehydration—running a marathon, for example, or walking all over Paris on the first day of your vacation, or spending five hours gardening in the summer heat and forgetting to take water breaks. Dehydration can lead to an electrolyte imbalance, meaning that levels of minerals that help cells function normally—sodium, calcium, and potassium—go out of kilter.

Inactivity, such as sitting too long in one position, can also bring on muscle cramps. Sometimes, they occur when you're just lying in bed, though no one's sure why.

To unkink and relax a tightened muscle, gently massage the area that's cramped, slowly stretch it, and then drink water or a sports drink to rehydrate. These herbal remedies will also help to soothe the ache.

Re-mineralize with nettle. Nettle is rich in minerals that can effectively alleviate cramping. Take one capsule or 30 drops of nettle tincture three times per day until the pain goes away. Mix the tincture with water, juice, or tea. A typical capsule dosage is between 300 and 450 milligrams.

Fight the ache with willow. For effective pain relief, take one-half teaspoon of willow bark tincture, mixed in juice, tea, or water. Willow bark contains salicin, an aspirin-like compound that naturally fights a wide variety of pain—from muscle cramps to headaches to arthritis. You can increase your dose to as much as five teaspoons if you choose white willow tincture, which has a lower salicin concentration.

Get relief with ginkgo. To improve blood flow in your limbs, and especially to knotted muscles, take one 80-milligram capsule of ginkgo (24 percent standardized extract) twice daily. Natural healers say ginkgo is an excellent choice for improving circulation.

Muscle Strains and Sprains

Even active, healthy women get their share of strains and sprains. An afternoon of digging up plants, playing tennis or golf, or even painting the house can leave you with a wrenched ankle or back, or with stiff, painful muscles the next morning.

A strain occurs when you pull or tear a muscle or tendon. A sprain happens when you pull or overstretch a ligament. In either case, pain and swelling are sure to occur.

With muscle injuries, quick treatment can make a real difference in healing by drastically reducing swelling, bruising, and further muscular damage. For first-aid, wrap some ice in a towel and hold it on the affected area. How long you keep it there depends on the size of the injured muscle. Small muscles, such as those in the calves and elbows, require 10- to 15-minute treatments. Large muscles, such as those in the back and thighs, require 20-minute treatments. Use ice up to six times a day, until the swelling goes down, bruising fades, and half the pain is gone.

After applying ice to the strain or sprain, incorporate these herbal healers.

Melt away pain with an herbal compress. Combine one to two teaspoons tincture of arnica or St. John's wort, and two tablespoons of cold water in a bowl. Soak a soft cloth in the mixture and apply the compress to the injured muscle to promote healing and to lessen the pain.

Rub on arnica oil. To combat bruising and swelling, apply arnica gel or oil to the affected muscle once a day for up to three days.

Stop swelling with bromelain. Herbal healers say this natural anti-inflammatory speeds healing of damaged tissue. Take 500 milligrams three times daily between meals until the pain subsides.

Pamper with herbal helpers. After a serious sprain, strain, or even broken bone has been treated by a doctor, enhance your long-term recovery with this two-part, skin-healing poultice-and-oil treatment. First, place one handful of fresh comfrey or plantain leaves and one-half cup water in a blender. Mix into a thick slush. Spread the poultice on a gauze pad, and place it, slush side down, over the area with the muscle strain or sprain. You can then cover the poultice with rolled cotton gauze to keep it in place. Leave the poultice on for up to one hour to reduce swelling. Both comfrey and plantain have skin-healing properties.

WOMEN ASK WHY

My husband uses a cayenne ointment for muscle pain. When he puts it on, he feels a burning sensation, but I've tried it, and I don't feel a thing. Does this mean it isn't going to work for me?

Cayenne ointment, also known as capsaicin cream, will work for you, but you may need to use more than your husband. Because everyone's skin is different, two people can have different reactions to the same cream. Perhaps your husband's skin is more sensitive to cayenne than yours is.

You should feel a warming or burning sensation when you apply cayenne ointment. That feeling tells you that capsaicin, the active ingredient in cayenne, is working. Capsaicin depletes substance P, a chemical made by your body that transmits pain messages from your nerves to your spinal cord. By disrupting those messages, you lessen pain.

Try using more of the ointment or use a stronger preparation. Most creams contain between .025 and .075 percent capsaicin. If you don't want to feel the burning sensation on your hands, wear disposable gloves when applying the cream. Don't use cayenne cream on broken or injured skin, and avoid getting it into your eyes.

Expert consulted
Jenny McFeely
Member of Britain's National Institute
  of Medical Herbalists
Professional member of the American
  Herbalists Guild
Scottsdale, Arizona

After the poultice, you can apply the following herbal healing oil: Combine two ounces of St. John's wort essential oil, one-eighth teaspoon lavender essential oil, eight drops marjoram essential oil, and two drops chamomile essential oil. Add this formula to about one-quarter cup of your favorite unscented massage oil or vegetable oil. Apply the oil to your skin over your injury as needed to enhance healing.

Nail Problems

When is the most likely time for a fingernail to split? Whenever it's most inconvenient, of course. You may be pulling on new panty hose, typing at a computer keyboard, or buttoning your coat as you rush out the door. Suddenly, a nail gives way and *rip*, your lovely manicure is ruined.

Fingernails can get brittle, weak, and dull when they're parched. Overexposure to household detergents, cold, heat, and wind causes nails to dry and break easily, leaving them with jagged edges, ragged cuticles, and cracked surrounding skin. Prolonged and repeated contact with water is also hazardous to your nails. Nails expand when they absorb water, then contract as the water evaporates. As water moves in and out of the nails, they weaken and crack. In addition, simply getting older can increase the chances that your nails will become thin and brittle.

In the 1950s, many women took calcium supplements or drank gelatin in hopes of growing stronger, longer nails that resisted chips and tears. These remedies don't work. Here's what today's natural healers and beauty experts recommend for growing stronger, longer nails that resist chips and tears.

Rub in herb-fortified castor oil. For ripped or dry nails, rub a drop of castor oil into the cuticle of each nail every day. Castor oil is thick and moisturizing, and it contains lots of vitamin E, so it's like food for your fingernails. An added bonus: It makes your nails shiny. Add a drop or two of skin-friendly carrot seed, lavender, or sandalwood essential oil to a two-ounce bottle of castor oil for improved results.

Dunk your nails in lavender and sandal-
wood. If your nails crack easily, strengthen them with an herbal soak. Combine two tablespoons jojoba oil with four drops each of lavender and sandalwood essential oils. Soak your nails in this mixture for 10 minutes. Then gently buff your nails to stimulate circulation and bring out a healthy shine.

Dip in horsetail. Nourish, condition, and protect dry, dull, brittle nails with a horsetail-comfrey soak. Horsetail is rich in silica, a substance that strengthens nails, according to experts on natural beauty. Comfrey has been used traditionally by herbal healers to soothe and mend damaged skin, and it will come to the aid of the cracked, dry skin around your nails. Combine one-half teaspoon of dried horsetail with one teaspoon of comfrey in a cup of boiling water. Steep for 15 to 20 minutes and let cool to a comfortable temperature. Then soak your nails in the mixture for 5 to 10 minutes. Repeat several times a week.

Nausea

What do bus fumes and intestinal parasites have in common? Both can make you feel sick to your stomach. So can nervousness, too much wine, or some powerful medications. Digestive infections, inner ear disorders, overindulgence in food (or drink), emotional stress, and toxic overloads on the liver can all contribute to nausea, too.

An effective way to treat nausea is to give it the heave-ho—by throwing up. Vomiting is your body's way of getting rid of something it doesn't want sticking around any longer.

But sometimes, whether you've vomited or not, nausea lingers, and your stomach churns and cramps. You may even feel feverish. Although most stomach upsets depart on their own within 24 hours, here are some herbs that offer fast, stomach-soothing relief.

Grab some ginger. Touted as the top herb for just about all types of stomach upsets, ginger relieves nausea as well as dizziness. Ginger in capsule form is strongest, so it has the greatest medicinal effect. The recommended dose is one to two capsules three times per day for as long as you feel under the weather. (A typical dosage is 550 milligrams per capsule.) Or make a hot drink: Buy fresh gingerroot and cut off a slice about as long as your index finger. Simmer in 16 ounces of hot water for 15 minutes, then drink. This recipe makes about two cups of ginger tea.

Improve digestion with dandelion. Ease nausea by aiding liver and digestive functions with this common backyard herb. Take one capsule, which typically contains about 520 milligrams, or 30 drops of dandelion root tincture with meals. If taking the tincture, squeeze it into one-quarter cup of water and sip it slowly until it's gone. Do this three times a day.

Boot out nausea with meadowsweet. A cup of meadowsweet tea can make that tummy feel better. Meadowsweet soothes inflammation, calming your system and reducing nausea. Use one tablespoon of the dried herb per cup of just-boiled water. Steep for 5 to 10 minutes before straining out the herb. Then take tiny sips.

Nicotine Withdrawal

Anyone who has ever tried to stop smoking, successfully or not, has paid a visit to hell.

Even though you've tossed the cigarettes, stashed the ashtrays, and announced to all your friends and family that cigarettes will never

THE HERBAL KITCHEN

"Goodbye to Those Low-Down, Tummy-Achin' Blues" Tonic

When that queasy, uneasy sensation of nausea unsettles your stomach, you want something that will bring relief quickly. Make a batch of this recipe and keep it on hand for moments of digestive distress, says Jenny McFeely, a member of Britain's National Institute of Medical Herbalists and a professional member of the American Herbalists Guild, who is from Scottsdale, Arizona. This mixture contains herbs that aid digestion and relax and calm the stomach.

¼ ounce black horehound tincture or extract

¼ ounce meadowsweet tincture or extract

¼ ounce anise tincture or extract

¼ ounce German chamomile tincture or extract

25 drops ginger tincture or extract

In a one-ounce or larger bottle with a dropper lid, mix the black horehound, meadowsweet, anise, and chamomile. Then add the ginger. Shake well. Take five to eight drops of the tonic as needed.

again touch your lips, you still want nicotine. In fact, you don't just want it. You *crave* it.

The truth is, cigarettes are just as addictive as cocaine or even heroin, and they're equally hard to ditch. More than one-third of people who try to stop smoking report significant withdrawal symptoms: irritability, anxiety, hunger, fatigue, dry mouth, headaches, insomnia, constipation, and, of course, the need for a cigarette.

But remember, nicotine withdrawal is only temporary. You *can* get through it. By contrast, a lifetime of smoking can lead to permanent problems: cancer, heart attacks, strokes, osteoporosis, fertility problems, and early menopause.

Women doctors say that exercise relieves irritability and anxiety and helps you avoid adding extra pounds when you quit smoking. Snacking on low-calorie foods such as carrot sticks, apples, and even sugarless gum helps, too. Herbs can also contribute to an easier, more peaceful transition to a smoke-free life. Consider these botanical options.

Clear your throat and calm your mind with a three-herb tea. Especially during your first few days without cigarettes, you may feel jittery and need to get rid of excess phlegm in your lungs. This anti-smoking herbal tea helps both problems. Blend equal amounts of dried chamomile, dried skullcap, and dried catnip, and then add two teaspoons of this mix per cup of just-boiled water. Steep up to 30 minutes, strain, and drink one-quarter cup four times per day. Chamomile is a gentle relaxant, as is skullcap, which has also been used to treat drug and alcohol addiction. Catnip, another relaxant, has been used traditionally for respiratory ailments.

Overcome nicotine withdrawal with oats and more. Calm withdrawal symptoms with this botanical formula suggested by natural healers. Combine one-half teaspoon each of the tinctures of valerian and skullcap, one teaspoon tincture of fresh oats, and one-half teaspoon each of the tinctures of St. John's wort and passion-flower. Take two to five dropperfuls of the mixture daily. Practitioners of Ayurvedic medicine have been recommending oats for at least 1,000 years to treat opium addiction. Recent studies have shown that a tincture made from oats can also help people stop smoking. The other herbs in this formula are calming and uplifting.

Reach for a cigarette substitute. If you miss holding a cigarette between your fingers or your lips, switch from cigarettes to a sweet stick of licorice root. Herbalists aren't sure how it works, but licorice root somehow satisfies oral cravings that people who are addicted to cigarettes seem to have. Don't substitute licorice candy, however, since it rarely contains real licorice.

LICORICE
Good for: digestion, coughs, and respiratory congestion

Night Sweats

Night sweats are nocturnal hot flashes. Unpredictable and uncomfortable, these symptoms of menopause can wake you from a sound sleep, drenched in perspiration.

Medical experts aren't sure what causes night sweats, but they seem to be linked to the hormonal changes that occur before and during menopause. It may be that your body's heat regulation system gets thrown off when hormones are in flux. Or it may be that hormonal changes irritate blood vessels and nerves, causing the blood vessels to overdilate, making you feel hot. In any case, night sweats interrupt sleep and can leave you irritable and depressed during the day.

For comfort, sleeping in all-cotton pajamas on all-cotton sheets is recommended. Synthetics or blends that trap body heat can trigger a night sweat. Also, keep a carafe of ice water on your nightstand to sip. During an episode, taking slow, deep breaths can help. And finally, you can turn to herbs.

Have a cool, herbal soak. Reduce the frequency and severity of night sweats by cooling off in an herbal bath before going to bed. Put the following essential oils into one-half cup of carrier oil, such as grapeseed, almond, or apricot: 4 drops of chamomile, 6 drops of lemon, and 10 drops of evening primrose. Then dump the mixture into a tub of comfortably warm—not hot—water. Soak in the bath long enough for the water to cool, usually about 20 minutes. Chamomile is said to relax the body, lemon cools and calms, and evening primrose aids hormonal balance.

Rely on motherwort. To subdue night sweats, herbalists suggest motherwort, a magnificent herbal ally for menopausal women. Dilute 5 to 15 drops of tincture of motherwort, made from fresh, flowering tops, in a little water or tea. Take as needed.

Act fast with sage. For quick results, stave off night sweats with garden sage. Make this tea in advance and keep it by your bedside: Add four heaping tablespoons of dried sage to one cup of hot water. Cover tightly and steep for four hours or more, then strain it. Sage is useful for menopause because of its estrogenic action and because it dries up perspiration.

Oily Hair

Contrary to popular belief, "problem" oily hair doesn't exist. The problem is not your hair. It's your scalp.

Oil on your scalp, just like the oil on your skin, comes from sebaceous glands. Attached to hair follicles, these sacs excrete sebum, a mixture of fatty acids, which prevents the scalp from drying out. Excess sebum weighs individual hairs down. As a consequence, your coif looks flat, dull, and lifeless.

Your hormones control how much sebum your sebaceous glands produce. That's why hair tends to look more oily during puberty, preg-

---

WOMAN TO WOMAN
No Need to Sweat Menopause

For Lorraine Banfi, 54, an insurance project manager in central New Jersey, the onset of menopause meant the beginning of misery. Night after night, she would awaken and find herself drenched in sweat, while during the day, she began having hot flashes so intense that she had to keep an oscillating fan under her desk to cool herself off. She tried everything she could think of before she finally found a solution to her problem. Here is her story.

About five years ago, I started going through menopause. Until then, I'd always been a sound sleeper, but suddenly, I began having trouble staying asleep. I'd wake up in cold sweats, damp and shivering, whether it was winter or summer, and my mattress and pillow always felt really uncomfortable.

I tried changing the quilt and blanket on my bed, but it didn't help. I tried to tire myself out more by reading and watching TV, but that didn't work either. I tried sleeping on a different bed, and I even moved to the sofa. Nothing helped.

A hormonal test at a gynecologist's office confirmed I was in menopause. The doctor put me on a mild birth control pill containing estrogen, but I immediately developed chronic headaches. They went on for two months. She replaced my first medication with a second one, but the headaches continued. Then she tried a third and a fourth. Finally, I'd had enough. I stopped taking medications. I decided just to live with the constant night sweats and hot flashes.

Luckily, I was still open to suggestions. I was taking a class in dried-flower arranging at the time, and a friend I'd made there told me about an herbalist who had helped her. I'd never used herbs before, but somehow the idea just seemed right to me. I decided to try them.

The herbalist gave me a formula containing black cohosh, chasteberry, oats, American ginseng, wild yam, and reishi. Mostly, it contained black cohosh and chasteberry. The black cohosh was supposed to keep my estrogen levels in balance. The chasteberry was for hot flashes and nervous tension.

Within six weeks, my hot flashes were gone, and to this day, I no longer have to keep a fan under my desk.

MAKE YOUR OWN HERBAL SHAMPOO

Some herbal and aromatherapy shampoos cost a pretty penny, but you can make a product that's just as good easily and inexpensively in your own home. This shampoo gently cleans yet doesn't strip away your hair's natural oils, and it doubles as an herbal body wash, says Mindy Green, a founding and professional member of the American Herbalists Guild, director of educational services for the Herb Research Foundation in Boulder, Colorado, and coauthor of *Aromatherapy: A Complete Guide to the Healing Art.*

To pick your herbs and essential oils, Green offers the following suggestions.

- Dry hair: Use the herbs orange peel, calendula, or comfrey. Use the essential oils sandalwood or rosewood.

- Oily hair: Use the herbs sage, lemongrass, burdock, or lemon peel. Use the essential oils lemongrass, patchouli, clary sage, cypress, or cedarwood.

- All types: Use the herbs lavender, chamomile, rosemary, or rose. Use the essential oils lavender, Roman chamomile, rosemary, or carrot seed.

- Dandruff: Use the herbs burdock, sage, or willow bark. Use the essential oils sage, geranium, juniper, cedarwood, or tea tree.

To make the shampoo, purchase an empty four-ounce shampoo bottle at a beauty supply store. (Limiting each batch to four ounces ensures freshness.) Using a funnel, pour in two ounces of an unscented shampoo base, which can be bought at a beauty supply or health food store. After choosing what herb or herbs you want to use, make two ounces of a strong infusion or decoction, depending on the herb. After the tea has cooled, strain it, and then combine it with the unscented shampoo. With an eyedropper, add 30 drops of your selected essential oils. (If you're using a teaspoon, 30 drops equals about one-quarter teaspoon.) Shake well before each use.

Make your own shampoo. If you can't locate a commercial shampoo that keeps your hair from looking oily, concoct your own. Just add four drops each of rosemary and lavender essential oils to two ounces of any unscented shampoo. Shake the mixture well, then wash your hair as usual. Start off with a quarter-size dollop, adjusting the amount to the length of your hair. Both rosemary and lavender essential oils control oiliness and add shine to your hair. Essential oils can irritate, so don't get this shampoo in your eyes. And if you notice any skin irritation, stop using it.

Improve your commercial shampoo with essential oils. If you love your store-bought shampoo, simply enhance it with this herbal formula: Dilute an eight-ounce bottle of shampoo by half with water and add about 20 drops of the essential oil of lavender, lemongrass, or patchouli. Regular shampooing with this mild, herb-rich formula will keep your oil glands under control.

Finish with an herbal rinse. To complete your hair-washing regimen, herbalists suggest this oil-fighting herbal rinse: Pour one pint of boiling water over one teaspoon each of the dried herbs burdock root, calendula flowers, chamomile flowers, lavender flowers, lemongrass, and sage leaves. Steep for about 30 minutes. Strain and add one tablespoon of vinegar. Pour this herbal mix over your scalp and hair as a final rinse after shampooing. For best results, don't rinse it out. The herbs discourage excess oil production, while the vinegar helps prevent dandruff.

nancy, and menopause, when hormonal changes accelerate sebum production.

Here are some herbal ways to keep excessive sebum production from masking your hair's natural beauty.

Oily Skin

Ah, the oily skin dilemma: Oil makes noses shine and chins glisten, but it also makes skin soft, supple, and less likely to wrinkle. So what's a woman with oily skin to do?

Blame excess oil on overeager sebaceous glands, tiny derricks that can sometimes pump out a little more lubrication than most women want or need. You may try to dispel excess oil with strong soaps and astringents. But natural beauty experts say they may be too harsh on your skin, and stripping too much oil away may simply signal your sebaceous glands to produce more.

Strike a healthy balance with these herbal remedies.

Gently conquer overactive oil glands with strawberry and lavender. Make oily skin feel clean and oil-free with a strawberry-lavender clay mask, herbal beauty experts suggest. Make the mask by combining one tablespoon of facial clay (available at health food stores), one tablespoon of witch hazel, one mashed strawberry, and one drop of lavender essential oil. Apply to your face, avoiding the area around your eyes. Leave it on for 10 to 15 minutes, then rinse with warm water. Strawberry helps normalize overactive oil glands, while lavender calms the central nervous system.

Steam open pores. To unclog pores and eliminate excess oil, steam your face with water and herbs at least once a week. Simmer three cups of water in a pan. Then add one heaping teaspoon each of chamomile, lemongrass, lavender, and rosemary. Remove from the heat and steep for five minutes. Set the pan in a place where you can comfortably sit next to it. Create a mini-sauna by covering the back of your head with a towel and tucking the ends around the pan. Hold your head about 12 inches away from the water. Make sure that the steam is not so hot that it feels uncomfortable. Be sure to keep your eyes closed so the oils don't sting. Remain in the steam for a few minutes, then come out to cool your face. Do this a few times.

The herbs will encourage your oil glands to function more normally.

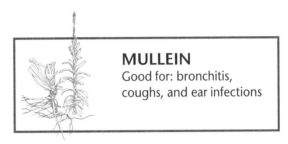

MULLEIN
Good for: bronchitis, coughs, and ear infections

Osteoporosis

A bump against the kitchen counter. A slip on an icy sidewalk. In your twenties, you might have hobbled away from such an encounter with nothing more than a colorful bruise on your hip. But in your fifties and beyond, even a minor bump or fall can break bones.

Why? Osteoporosis. It leaves bones weak, brittle, and porous. It may show no outward symptoms for years—which explains why more than 25 million Americans, among them many postmenopausal women, don't even know they have osteoporosis until they sustain a fracture. Women are at particular risk after menopause because production of the female hormone estrogen sharply declines. Estrogen helps bones absorb and retain calcium.

Bone loss actually starts much earlier in a woman's life. After age 35, she'll lose a little every year. In 20 years, she'll be down by 10 to 20 percent. You can slow that loss down, or even add some bone, with regular exercise, calcium supplements, and herbs. Women medical experts recommend at least 30 minutes of weight-bearing exercise (such as jogging or weight lifting) every day as well as walking at least 30 minutes three times a week. In addition, supplement your diet with at least 1,200 milligrams of calcium and 300 to 500 milligrams of magnesium daily. Then, complete your anti-osteoporosis strategy with these helpful herbs.

Maximize calcium intake with gentian. Ensure that calcium is properly absorbed from food and vitamin supplements by taking one capsule of gentian root before each meal (a typical capsule is 550 milligrams). This herb prompts stomach acids to effectively break down calcium so that it can be absorbed more completely.

Reduce your risk with horsetail. Horsetail is among the richest plant sources of silicon, a mineral that helps prevent osteoporosis and can be used to treat bone fractures, according to French studies. Natural healers suggest taking up to nine 350-milligram capsules of horsetail per day, but consult with a holistic practitioner to find the proper dose for you.

You can also take horsetail in tea form by adding about one tablespoon of dried horsetail and one teaspoon of sugar to each cup of water you use. Bring to a boil in a pan, then simmer for about three hours. Strain the leaves. Allow the tea to cool before drinking. (The sugar pulls more silicon from the herb.)

Appreciate avocados. For an added bone fortifier, sprinkle black pepper generously on avocados. Black pepper contains four anti-osteoporosis compounds. Avocado is loaded with bone-healthy vitamin D and heart-healthy vitamin E. Try mashing an avocado into calcium-rich nonfat cottage cheese or yogurt and sprinkling black pepper on top.

REAL-LIFE SCENARIO
Stopping a Family Disease Before It Starts

Sandra, 42, watched her mother gradually deteriorate with osteoporosis until she needed a wheelchair. Sandra is determined to have a healthier future for herself, so she makes sure she gets plenty of calcium: She drinks three glasses of milk each day, eats yogurt for snacks or lunch, and takes a calcium supplement with dinner. Even better, she now has a great excuse for indulging in her favorite food: cheese. The challenge is that all these dairy products are making her gain weight. Gas and constipation have also become annoyances. Are there better ways for her to keep this disease at bay?

Yes, there are. Sandra's efforts are commendable, but her preventive strategy is missing the most important bone-boosting therapy of all: weight-bearing exercise.

Weight-bearing exercise—such as walking, cross-country skiing, dancing, and climbing stairs—is so-named because it forces you to move or support either your body weight or added resistance weight, such as dumbbells, to build strength. It prevents osteoporosis by stimulating the body to make new bone.

There's one thing that Sandra is doing right: She's making an effort to get enough calcium through diet and supplements. She could, however, make better nutritional choices than high-fat, hard-to-digest dairy products. She might, for

Overweight

Let's admit it: If there really were a magic weight-loss pill, we'd all stock our shelves with it—and own stock in the company that makes it. There isn't, and we don't. Natural healers and conventional practitioners alike are still giving the same old advice: The most effective natural solution for unwanted pounds is still a combination of healthy diet and regular exercise.

example, switch from cow's milk to calcium-fortified soy milk. Soy milk won't cause gas or constipation, and it offers an extra bonus: It contains compounds, called phytoestrogens, that may actually strengthen bones. Other calcium-rich foods are often overlooked because they bear no resemblance at all to dairy products. They include canned salmon or sardines (with the bones included), and dark green leafy vegetables such as collards, turnip greens, mustard greens, and dandelion greens.

Taking a daily calcium supplement (with vitamin D and boron to ensure absorption) is a good idea, but it's important that Sandra take it before going to bed and not at dinnertime, since some common foods can prevent absorption. Because it is better absorbed at night, a bedtime dose may also help to limit calcium loss from her bones while she sleeps.

Once Sandra enters menopause, she should talk to her doctor about hormone-replacement therapy, which has been shown to significantly lower a woman's risk of developing osteoporosis. But she doesn't have to wait until then to have her bone strength, or density, measured. Having what's called a DEXA scan now will give her a basis for comparison later.

Expert consulted
Cynthia Phillips, N.D.
Naturopathic physician
Institute of Complementary Medicine
Seattle

Eat more foods high in fiber, such as fruits, vegetables, beans, potatoes, and whole grains. Fiber gives you the feeling of being full and stabilizes blood sugar levels. In addition, make time for at least 30 minutes of aerobic exercise five to seven days a week. Walking counts, as does any other activity that gets your heart pumping faster and your lungs working harder, including running, bicycling, swimming, or taking an aerobics class. Remember to check with your doctor before starting any exercise program.

That said, don't discount herbs. Chosen and used with care, they can give a sensible weight-loss program an added advantage. Sometimes, they may even make all the difference between success and failure.

Rev up your metabolism with green tea. For a safe weight-loss herb, herbalists suggest drinking a cup of green tea with a meal two or three times per day. Or take two 170-milligram capsules three times per day. Green tea contains caffeine and theobromine, both of which are stimulants. "So why don't I just drink a cup of coffee?" you might ask. Green tea has nutritional advantages that coffee doesn't, including vitamin C and flavonoids, potent antioxidants that reduce the risk of illnesses such as heart disease and colon cancer.

If you're trying to cut back on caffeine, though, don't have more than two cups of green tea per day.

Sprinkle cayenne on your food. If you're trying to lose weight, call on cayenne pepper (also known as red pepper), which raises your metabolic rate and stimulates thirst. If you fill up on water instead of food, you'll take in fewer calories and gain less weight. Add a dash of cayenne pepper to your food several times per day. In research conducted at Oxford Polytechnic Institute in England, dieters who added one teaspoon of cayenne pepper and one teaspoon of mustard to every meal raised their metabolic rates by as much as 25 percent.

Shed pounds with a five-star herb formula. Here's a gentle blend that can help you to lose pounds and improve your metabolism.

stores. Take one-half to one tea-spoon three times per day. Hold your nose before you drink, how-ever, because this isn't the most pleasant-tasting of concoctions.

Nettle is loaded with minerals, which help maintain overall health. Dandelion aids the liver in secreting bile, which helps break down fats. Bladderwrack is a folk remedy for being overweight. Guggul helps normalize thyroid function, which is sometimes disturbed in overweight people. Schizandrin, the active in-gredient in schisandra berry, stimu-lates metabolism.

Perimenopause

For women in their midforties to late fifties, perimenopause can be a frustrating and confusing gray zone. You're on the brink of menopause—as if you're standing at the very edge of a diving board, about to leap in—yet you're still not completely fin-ished with menstruation.

Usually, the first signs of peri-menopause are irregular or shorter menstrual cycles. The female hor-mone estrogen (and sometimes progesterone) starts to cycle at lower levels. The uterus reacts by shedding its lining early or off-schedule. In addition, some women experience symptoms that are similar to those of menopause: hot flashes, night sweats, insomnia, vaginal dryness, heart palpita-tions, depression, anxiety, and forgetfulness.

As a result, many botanical solutions recom-mended for perimenopause by herbalists and naturopaths are the same as those suggested for

Blend the following tinctures in an eight-ounce or larger bottle: one ounce of nettle, one ounce of dandelion leaf, one ounce of bladderwrack, two ounces of guggul, and two ounces of schisandra berry. All are available at health food menopause. Let these herbs assist you during this transitional time in life.

Rely on black cohosh. For relief from most of the discomforts this time of life may bring you, especially hot flashes, anxiety, and vaginal dryness, try black cohosh. The recommended dosage is a 40-milligram capsule (containing a standardized extract of 2.5 to 2.6 percent triterpene glycosides) two to four times daily. Clinical studies bear out that it can relieve many perimenopausal symptoms.

Balance hormones with chasteberry. To even out hormonal imbalances at perimenopause, natural healers recommend chasteberry (also known as vitex). If you have irregular periods, take a dropperful of chasteberry tincture in a small glass of water or juice two or three times per day for six to eight weeks. This shrub has been studied extensively and has been proven to relieve hot flashes, dizziness, and menstrual irregularities. Chasteberry influences the pituitary gland to slow down secretion of the hormone prolactin, which helps to normalize irregular menstrual cycles.

Enjoy soy. To fight hot flashes, balance estrogen, and protect against uterine and breast cancer, take 50 milligrams of soy-extract isoflavones two or three times per day. In nations where women eat soy products regularly, perimenopausal symptoms are less severe.

REAL-LIFE SCENARIO

She Found an Herbal Sugar Substitute

Barbara, age 43, has been trying to lose the same 30 pounds since junior high school. She blames her weight problems on her sweet tooth. She loves candy and cookies and seems to crave something sugary several times a day. Lately, she has discovered stevia, a super-sweet herb that comes in dried or liquid form. She adds it to everything—iced tea, hot tea, cereal, baked goods. Has Barbara found the answer to her craving for sugar?

The best thing Barbara can do for herself is to replace her sugary treats with healthier food and drink choices that don't need sweetening.

Of course, that's the sort of advice anyone on any street corner would give her—and it's boring. Like most people, every now and then Barbara needs to treat herself to something so sweet it's naughty.

That's where stevia comes in. Stevia, an herb imported into the United States from Paraguay, is as sweet as sugar but has no calories. Compare that to the 16 calories contained in just one teaspoon of cane or beet sugar. In the candy and cookies that Barbara favors, the amount of calories is huge. And worse, calories from sugar don't have much nutritional value. They're what's known as empty calories.

Using stevia instead of sugar in her baked goods and other sweet treats still doesn't give Barbara much nutritional value, but she's cutting out quite a few calories. And what she may not know is that stevia doesn't promote tooth decay, so she's doing her smile a favor as well. Barbara has made a good start, and she's benefiting from her switch to stevia in more ways than she probably realizes.

By modifying her diet and substituting stevia for sugar, she will probably lose a good bit of the 30 pounds she has been carrying around since junior high school. And she'll be able to enjoy herself while she's doing it.

Expert consulted
Emily Kane, N.D.
Naturopathic physician
Juneau, Alaska

PMS

Some women jokingly refer to premenstrual syndrome (PMS) as pity-me-syndrome. But PMS is no joke, and it's relief—not pity—that women with it seek.

The monthly discomfort of PMS strikes 8 out of every 10 women. Some weep without reason. Others blow their stacks or experience unstoppable food cravings. Still others complain of bloating, headaches, and acne breakouts. All told, PMS has more than 150 possible symptoms.

The cause behind PMS is still unknown. Some scientific studies indicate that some women with PMS possess below-normal levels of serotonin, a mood-regulating brain chemical. Another theory links PMS to fluctuating levels of estrogen and progesterone, both female hormones.

With its many symptoms, PMS isn't a simple condition to relieve. Top herbalists work with women to create customized PMS formulas to match their specific needs. Generally, they choose herbs that help balance hormones, stop mood swings, and improve liver function, which helps your body to eliminate excess hormones more effectively. Over a period of months, these herbal treatments can help your body function in a healthier way and free you from many of the challenges PMS can offer. Here are some herbs to try.

Chase away PMS with chasteberry. Chasteberry (also known as vitex) can give you a great head start on coping with PMS. To make a tea, use one teaspoon of the dried herb per cup of boiling water. Steep for 20 minutes, strain, then drink up to three cups per day. Studies show that chasteberry extract relieves end-of-cycle symptoms in women more effectively than vitamin B$_6$, a time-honored PMS remedy. Herbal experts say chasteberry seems to work by elevating levels of progesterone, the female hormone that rules the second half of the menstrual cycle.

Deflate bloating with yarrow. When PMS causes your abdomen to swell, reverse bloating with yarrow, herbal healers suggest. Combine one-half part dried yarrow and one part dried chasteberry to make a tea. Then use one teaspoon of this mix per cup of boiling water. Steep 20 minutes, strain, and sip up to three cups daily. A mild diuretic, yarrow also stimulates the liver, which helps balance hormones.

Pacify PMS moods with aromatherapy. To fend off anger or anxiety, rely on aromatherapy to put you in a better mood. For anger, dab two drops of rose and three drops of sandalwood essential oils on a handkerchief and smell it. For anxiety, try sniffing the scent of sandalwood, ylang-ylang, or orange blossom essential oil.

NETTLE
Good for: allergy and hay fever symptoms

Poison Ivy, Poison Oak, and Poison Sumac

"Three leaves, leave it be." Maybe your grandpa taught you this warning the first time you hiked the woods with him. It's good advice if you don't want to leave the woods itchy. That old-time saying reminds you to avoid contact with poison ivy. But you should also steer clear of poison oak and poison sumac.

Poison ivy thrives in ankle-deep ground cover, especially on the East Coast. Poison oak is more common to the West Coast. Poison sumac is a shrub or small tree with white berries common in swampy areas of the East Coast.

A few lucky people aren't allergic to urushiol, the thick, oily substance in the resin of these plants that provokes that annoying, itchy rash. Most of us, however, aren't so fortunate. Even indirect contact—such as handling clothing or shoes that have brushed against a poison plant or petting a dog or cat that just rolled in a poison ivy patch—can raise those itchy blisters on your skin.

This allergic reaction can also make you feel nauseated, tired, fuzzy-headed, and feverish. In severe cases, it can lead to unrelenting itching and infection, and sometimes, the rash even spreads to the face or eyes. If you develop such a severe rash, see your doctor—you may need a cortisone shot.

Milder cases respond well to herbal remedies. Before reaching for herbal relief, however, first carefully remove urushiol from your skin, advise women medical experts. As soon as possible, wash thoroughly with soap or a strong detergent. (Fels Naptha soap works very well.) Remove all clothing and wash it. Then try these itch-stopping, rash-relieving herbal remedies.

Be prepared with grindelia. Before setting out on a hiking trip through the woods, plan ahead by packing a tincture of grindelia (also called gumweed) in your backpack. Immediately after brushing up against a poisonous plant, wipe your exposed skin with grindelia tincture.

Nix the itch with an herbal paste. If you're already itching and sporting an oozing rash, soothe your skin with an herbal paste. Combine two tablespoons of grindelia or jewelweed tincture and two tablespoons of comfrey tincture with one-eighth cup distilled water. Stir the liquid ingredients into one-quarter cup of colloidal oatmeal (available in drugstores) or one to two tablespoons of bentonite clay until you form a paste. If colloidal oatmeal is not available, grind whole oatmeal in a coffee mill or blender. Apply to the affected skin. These herbs calm the itch and discourage oozing. Allow the paste to dry on your skin and leave it on until you bathe.

Halt swelling with echinacea. Herbalists say you can soothe the inflammation of a poison-plant rash with an echinacea wash. Just mix one part echinacea tincture in three parts water. Use the wash on affected skin several times per day. German research shows that echinacea helps reduce inflammation when applied externally.

Psoriasis

Television advertisements used to call it the heartbreak of psoriasis—and, indeed, the red rashes and silvery scales brought on by this skin condition are both unsightly and uncomfortable. Natural healers say the best way to soothe psoriasis is with a combination of remedies that work on the outside surface of the skin as well as others that work from inside of you.

In psoriasis, skin cells grow at an abnormal rate, often 1,000 times faster than normal. These cells pile up in clumps that look like silvery scales. Although unsightly red patches and scales can appear anywhere on your skin, they usually show up on your scalp, the backs of your ears, your elbows, or behind your knees.

Pinpointing the reason for this rapid cell division can be difficult, but medical experts say people with psoriasis usually have high levels of polyamine, a toxic amino acid that forms as a result of poor digestion. Stress also plays a role. More than one-third of people with psoriasis say their initial outbreak occurred within a month of a very stressful event. Outbreaks can also be provoked by injuries, infections, or a change of season. This skin condition may be inherited but is not contagious.

The first steps in psoriasis relief? Stop using soap. It will irritate sensitive skin. And try to get out in the sun for about an hour per day. Exposure to ultraviolet light slows down the abnormal growth of skin cells.

Natural healers also recommend specific herbs that soothe skin and improve liver function. They believe that when the liver can't process the toxins, hormones, fats, and other substances in the bloodstream completely, some toxins are sent to the skin to be eliminated. If these toxins irritate the skin, it worsens a psoriasis outbreak. Here are some ways to soothe psoriasis, on the surface and from deep within.

Cleanse with healing herbs. Instead of using soap, try this herbal cleanser especially designed for dry skin and psoriasis. Blend two ounces of aloe vera gel, one teaspoon of vegetable oil, one teaspoon of glycerin, one-half teaspoon of grapefruit seed extract, eight drops of sandalwood essential oil, and four drops of rosemary essential oil. Shake well before each use. Apply with cotton balls to the affected skin areas, then rinse off. This cleanser fights inflammation and heals the irritation that develops as outer layers of dry skin flake off.

Rally 'round your liver with milk thistle or yellow dock. A tincture of yellow dock or milk thistle will boost liver function, natural healers note. Take 30 to 60 drops of either in water, juice, or herbal tea, two or three times per day for up to nine months. These traditional skin healers help the liver filter out toxins that irritate sensitive skin.

POISON PLANTS
AND THEIR ANTIDOTES

If poison ivy, oak, or sumac caresses your exposed skin while you're hiking and you're miles from washing facilities, search the roadsides and woodland edges for jewelweed.

Scientists have discovered that jewelweed contains a chemical called lawsone. This substance blocks the action of urushiol, the plant resin that causes the allergic reaction. If applied quickly after contact with a poisonous plant, lawsone locks out urushiol and prevents rashes from developing.

Grab a bunch of jewelweed (leaves and stems), crush it into a ball in your hands, and rub your skin with its juice, says Ellen Evert Hopman, a professional member of the American Herbalists Guild and author of *Tree Medicine, Tree Magic.* If you can find them, use the reddish protuberances, which are actually rootlets, on the lower stem of jewelweed. These may contain the highest concentrations of lawsone. Squeeze the liquid out of the rootlets onto a tissue or directly onto the rash. It may take a few plants to get enough of the liquid.

Jewelweed. In moist, shaded areas, this tall plant often grows alongside of poison ivy, since both plants are prolific weeds. Unlike poison ivy, however, jewelweed can't grow in dry areas. Because jewelweed may have poison ivy neighbors, be sure to carefully choose leaves that are farthest from any nearby poison ivy plants. This will eliminate any possible exposure to the ivy's irritating oils. Look for the orange-flowered variety, not the yellow. The orange flowers bloom from June to September.

Poison ivy. This woody plant grows as a shrub or as a climbing or creeping vine. The plant has three shiny leaves—the middle leaf is bigger than the other two—connected to one stem. The leaves are reddish when they first appear in spring, green in the summertime, and various shades of red, orange, yellow, or bronze in the fall. Poison ivy leaves can be up to 10 inches long, and the plant's tiny yellow-green flowers grow in clusters. It prefers growing in rich soil under good light and has an affinity for rail fences, but this tough plant will grow practically anywhere.

Poison oak. Poison oak can reach 6½ feet tall, and its stems are slender and woody. Like poison ivy, the plant is identified by three leaves. But unlike ivy, the leaves have rounded tips. The foliage resembles oak leaves. Small white flowers with five petals grow in clusters.

Poison sumac. This is a tall shrub or small tree with 6 to 12 leaflets arranged in pairs, with one single leaflet at the end of each branch. The clustered flowers start out as small and yellow-green, but they evolve into white-green fruits that hang on loose clusters four to eight inches long. Nonpoisonous sumac grows red fruits with cone-shaped heads.

Puffy Eyes

Blame baggy, under-eye pouches on too little sleep—or too many tears. Allergies, salty foods, and hormonal changes during the menstrual cycle can also prompt your body to collect and retain fluid under your eyes.

Whatever the cause, walking around with puffy eyes is no picnic. Wraparound sunglasses help—when you're out in the sun. So do cover-up concealer creams—as long as they're not so light that they actually attract attention to your eyes. But instead of hiding them, try these gentle herbal solutions to deflate those under-eye pouches.

Ease away puffiness with fennel. If you're prone to puffy eyes, have this cool-comfort remedy ready to use. Pour a cup of boiling water over two teaspoons of fennel seeds and cover. Let steep, then put the whole pot in the refrigerator overnight. In the morning, strain the cooled tea, which should smell like licorice.

Cut paper towels into patches slightly larger than your eyes and soak them in the cool fennel tea. Lie down with your head elevated on a pillow. Cover your closed eyes with the patches. Re-wet the patches whenever they warm up. Within 15 minutes, your eyes should look and feel better. This mixture lasts four days when stored in the refrigerator.

Go with chamomile for quick relief. Rely on chamomile tea bags to unpuff those eyes, natural beauty experts say. Just close your eyes and lay wet, chilled chamomile tea bags over them for 10 to 20 minutes. Chamo-

Barb Wallace, a 33-year-old mother of two young sons, lives in Brooks, Alberta, a bitterly cold Canadian province where the frigid, long-lasting winters were taking a painful toll on her sinuses. Fed up with over-the-counter cough syrups, nasal sprays, and decongestant capsules, she looked to natural remedies for relief. Here's her story.

I grew up in Brooks. It's a town of about 10,000 people best known for its clean water, oil companies, and dinosaur fossils. Of course, it's cold—winters seem to arrive early and stay late—but it's a family town I really enjoy.

By October of every year, the temperature has dropped and my nasal passages get so stuffed up that I get pressure headaches in my forehead—not to mention ringing in my ears. My eyes get dry and sore, and I can feel mucus roll down my throat. My medicine cabinet used to be filled with all kinds of cough syrups, nasal sprays, and sinus capsules, both over-the-counter and prescription. It seemed like I tried them all, but I didn't like the side effects. I also didn't like the idea of putting chemicals into my body.

Then, one day, I was reading about herbs and came across echinacea as a good treatment for head colds, sinusitis, and the flu. I was very disbelieving. How could anything work that well? But I decided to consult a naturopathic physician anyway. Her name is Angela Stengler. She told me to take echinacea capsules. It was like a miracle. Within four hours of taking the first capsules, I definitely felt improvement, and with no side effects.

Now, I take echinacea, along with bioflavonoids, whenever I first start to feel sinus pressure or a sore throat coming on. If I catch it quickly, by the next day, I feel 90 percent better. I know this is not an herb to take every day, like a multivitamin. It should only be taken when I feel symptoms coming on. I also learned that sugar from soda aggravates sinus conditions and sore throats, so even though I love drinking Pepsi, I stay off it while I'm taking echinacea.

All in all, I've had great success with herbal remedies.

mile gently constricts blood vessels, which may help minimize puffiness. Don't use this remedy if you're allergic to pollen. You may react to the pollen-rich flower heads found in chamomile.

Restore bright eyes with dandelion. Gently flush excess fluid—which can cause under-eye puffiness—out of your body by drinking a cup or two of dandelion tea per day. To make the tea, use one teaspoon of dried dandelion leaf and one teaspoon of dried dandelion root per cup of boiling water. Steep in a teapot or covered pan for 10 minutes. Then strain and sip. Dandelion acts as a cleansing diuretic that reduces water retention. If you have gallbladder disease, don't use dandelion preparations without your doctor's approval.

Sinusitis

Sometimes, your body's air-filtration system goes on the fritz. Viruses, pollen, or polluted air can irritate and inflame the delicate mucous membranes lining your nasal passages, cutting off drainage from your sinus cavities.

The result is pressure and r in across your forehead and around your eyes and nose. You develop a stuffed-up, can't-breathe feeling. Sometimes, headaches occur. Your eyes may become red, itchy, and scratchy. If infection sets in, you may also develop a fever and experience nasal discharge.

Some women come down with

sinusitis only occasionally. For others, it's a painful, chronic condition. Along with decongestants, antibiotics are usually prescribed if an infection has flared up. If you have a fever, a pus-like nasal discharge, or persistent pain, see your doctor. If your symptoms are less severe, consider the following botanical remedies, recommended by top herbalists.

Unclog with goldenseal. Soothe inflamed mucous membranes fast with goldenseal. Try 10 to 25 drops of goldenseal tincture mixed in water as often as five times per day. Goldenseal contains two active compounds that fight infection. Use this herb only until your sinus inflammation has cleared. It is not meant for long-term use.

Inhale congestion-clearing eucalyptus. Create a sinus-soothing steam with eucalyptus essential oil, herbalists suggest. Heat up some water on the stove until it boils, then pour it into a bowl. Add a couple drops of eucalyptus essential oil. Drape a towel over your head, and keeping your face about 12 inches away from the water, breathe in the steam from the bowl for about five minutes. The humidity of the steam and the action of the essential oil work to loosen mucus and help you to breathe freely.

Tame sinus headaches with eyebright. To ease the pain of a sinus headache, herbalists recommend taking five milligrams of eyebright tincture, mixed in water, every four to six hours until the pain and infection disappear. This grasslike herb combines anti-inflammatory powers with an astringent action. Besides subduing sinus headaches, eyebright also helps to dry up congestion and runny noses.

PEPPERMINT
Good for: preventing indigestion and treating bad breath, gas, and nausea

Sore Throats

Marathon chats. Cigarette smoke. Cheering at a football game. A cold. A cough. An allergy. Any—and all—of these can leave your throat raw, scratchy, and inflamed.

Sore throats happen when the mucous membrane lining your airways dries out. The result? It hurts to swallow.

If you develop a sore throat with a fever—and no other cold or allergy symptoms—you may have a strep infection, which requires medical attention. Should your doctor determine that you have strep throat, she will probably prescribe antibiotics.

But for routine sore throats, here's what nature has to offer.

Gargle away infection with soothing herbs. If your throat is infected and full of mucus, gargle with a tea made from the dried herb sage, thyme, goldenseal, echinacea, or myrrh. Take a teaspoonful of your chosen herb, add eight ounces of boiling water, let it steep in a covered container for 10 minutes, and strain. Allow it to cool to a comfortable temperature, then gargle with it as often as necessary. These herbs fight infection and reduce inflammation.

Suck on slippery elm. For dry, scratchy, sore throats, slippery elm lozenges can supply a steady stream of relief. Slippery elm is rich in soothing mucilage, which means it creates a little healthy mucus to help you expel whatever irritants are making you cough, and it protects irritated mucous membranes. It also acts as a mild cough suppressant.

Sip marshmallow tea. To soothe and moisten a dry, irritated throat during the day, sip on marshmallow root tea. To make the tea, put one-quarter cup dried, chopped marshmallow root in a glass or ceramic jar. Then pour one pint of room-temperature water over it. Cover the jar and allow the herb to steep overnight. In the

THE HERBAL KITCHEN
Soothing Sore Throat Tea

Calm an irritated throat with this soothing, easy-to-make herbal tea, created by Angela Stengler, N.D., a naturopathic physician and herbal author in Oceanside, California.

1   piece fresh gingerroot, 5 inches long and ½–1½ inches thick
1   tablespoon dried licorice root
6   cups water
20   drops echinacea tincture
20   drops goldenseal tincture
1   tablespoon honey

Chop the fresh gingerroot into fine pieces or shred it using a cheese grater. Put the ginger, licorice root, and water into a saucepan. Bring to a boil. Cover the pan with a lid and simmer on low for 20 minutes. Remove from the stove, strain. Pour into a teacup, adding the echinacea and goldenseal tinctures. Add the honey. Drink one cup every three hours to relieve sore throat pain.

Ginger can help reduce pain and inflammation. Licorice provides a pleasant taste and is thought to aid the immune system against viruses. Echinacea boosts the body's immune system. Goldenseal is used to fight bacteria. Honey is a sweet-tasting antibacterial and antimicrobial.

morning, strain and add four teaspoons of honey to the liquid. Sip one-quarter to one-half cup of tea at a time throughout the day. The mixture is only good for one day, so drink as much as you can in one day and dispose of the rest.

Stress

Sometimes, the smallest thing can unleash feelings of tension and stress: the alarm clock that didn't go off. A cup of coffee spilling into your lap. Bumper-to-bumper traffic. Work deadlines. Family demands. The dog that overturns the trash can. The list is endless.

Simply put, stress is any pressure that disrupts the regular rhythms of your life and emotions. This pressure can come in the form of a physical complaint, such as a cold or an aching knee joint. It can be purely emotional, like worry over a pressing deadline or anger about a romantic breakup. Or it can be an assault from without, such as a noisy mob or a frightening thunderstorm.

Any of these stresses can leave you feeling depressed, irritable, edgy, or anxious. Sustained stress can elevate blood pressure, weaken your immune system, trigger headaches and backaches, and raise your risk for a host of serious disorders, such as heart disease.

Knowing healthy ways to unshackle stress's grip gives you more control over life's expected—and unexpected—challenges. Relaxation techniques, deep breathing, physical activity, getting enough sleep, and eating well can all help you resist its ravages. Herbs can play a vital role, too. Botanical remedies won't make stress magically disappear, but they can be a helpful addition to your personal stress-management plan.

Create serenity with an herbal formula. If you face a seriously stressful situation, you can ease your body and your mind quickly with this blend. Combine two parts each of the tinctures of skullcap and valerian plus one part each of tinctures of motherwort, chamomile, and mugwort. Take a teaspoon of this blend as needed.

Skullcap and valerian are traditional stress-relief herbs. Chamomile aids in digestion to prevent stomach upsets, mugwort is a gentle sedative, and motherwort helps you to relax and calms heart palpitations.

Unwind with a lavender bath. If you've had an especially brutal, stressful day, help ensure a good night's sleep by first soaking in a lavender bath. Essential oils aren't soluble in bathwater, but they do dissolve in milk, so add one to five drops of lavender essential oil to one-half cup of milk. Pour this mix into a tub of comfortably warm water and relax. Make sure you select the *Lavandula angustifolia* species of this herb, which is noted for its floral, relaxing scent.

Bust stress with aromatherapy. To elevate your mood when stress strikes, tailor the aroma of essential oils to your personal needs. Concoct a take-along bottle of stress-busting smelling salts by combining one tablespoon of coarse rock salt with six drops of essential oil in a bowl. Mix well. Transfer to a small, dark glass bottle with a tight-fitting lid. When you feel stressed, open the bottle and gently fan the fragrance with your hand toward your nose. Then sit back, close your eyes, and breathe deeply.

Which essential oils should you choose? For tension, try lavender and orange; for anger and irritability, use bergamot and chamomile; for anxiety, try cedar and ylang-ylang.

Stress-proof with Siberian ginseng. To protect your body from the effects of stress, herbalists recommend taking one-half to three-quarters teaspoon of Siberian ginseng tincture three times per day. Take the herb daily for six weeks, followed by a two-week break, then resume for as long as necessary. Siberian ginseng contains at least 18 different hormonelike saponins that botanists say fight stress and fatigue.

ROSEMARY
Good for: preventing migraines and treating congestion and fever

Stretch Marks

Many women associate stretch marks with pregnancy and weight gain, but other factors can stretch the skin's elastic tissue to the max, leaving behind those unmistakable lines.

Exercises that bulk up muscle can do it. So can prolonged use of high-potency cortisone creams and other corticosteroid medications.

Stretch marks initially appear as pinkish or purplish lines on the breasts, abdomen, buttocks, thighs, and sometimes the arms. Gradually, they lighten or turn white and shiny.

Once you have these scarlike marks, they stick around for a lifetime. Moisturizers, wrinkle creams, and massages won't make them vanish, say medical experts. But you can take steps to avoid getting more stretch marks, with good nutrition, regular exercise, and the following herbal remedy.

Rub on skin balm. Minimize or even avoid stretch marks before they happen by rubbing this herbal balm into skin that you know will be stretched (such as on your belly early in pregnancy). Combine four ounces of almond oil or a blend of almond and olive oil with a few drops of lavender essential oil and an ounce or more of calendula infused oil.

The best application method is to rub this herbal balm all over your belly daily, from the top of your pubic bone to the bottom of your rib cage. The oils and herbs will help keep the skin supple and help it stretch without leaving stretch marks. Lavender essential oil is soothing and

Both lavender essential oil and the gel of the aloe vera plant can reduce inflammation and soothe tender, sunburned skin. Combine the healing and cooling powers of both in this sunburn spray created by Mindy Green, a founding and professional member of the American Herbalists Guild, director of educational services for the Herb Research Foundation in Boulder, Colorado, and coauthor of *Aromatherapy: A Complete Guide to the Healing Art*.

In a small spritzer bottle, mix together 50 drops (about one-half teaspoon) of lavender essential oil, four ounces of aloe vera juice, one teaspoon of vitamin E oil, and one tablespoon of vinegar. (Lavender essential oil, aloe vera juice, and vitamin E oil are all available at health food stores.)

Shake well before each use. Spray as often as needed to reduce sunburn pain. Store the bottle in the refrigerator to chill the spray and enhance the cooling sensation on the skin.

antimicrobial, while calendula contains skin-healing properties.

Sunburn

Whether you're on the golf course, at the beach, or working in your garden, the sun's ultraviolet rays initially feel invitingly warm on your skin. But overexposure to the sun can leave unprotected skin painfully tender, red, swollen, and even blistery.

What's going on? Medical experts say that the blood vessels near your skin's surface dilate in response to being exposed to too much sun. Anyone can get a sunburn, but fair-skinned women and those with blonde, red, or brown hair are at the greatest risk for sun-related skin damage. Some medications can make you more sensitive to the sun, too.

Minimize sunburns by heeding these rules:

Avoid direct sunlight from 10:00 A.M. to 3:00 P.M., when the sun's harmful rays are the strongest. And stay covered with a brimmed hat, longer shorts, long-sleeve shirts, and sunglasses. Apply sunblock with a sun protection factor (SPF) of 15 or higher.

If your sunburn is so severe that you have blisters, a fever, chills, or severe pain, you could have sun poisoning. Get medical attention immediately. These symptoms can also indicate the possibility of heat exhaustion or heatstroke.

For routine sunburn, try these herbal offerings to relieve the pain, reduce the swelling, and hasten the healing.

Make aloe your ally. For immediate treatment of minor sunburn, herbalists suggest you cut or snap off a leaf from a mature aloe plant. Cut it down its length and squeeze out the transparent gel from inside the leaf directly onto your sunburned skin. Aloe forms a coating on the surface of your skin that helps prevent dehydration from the inside out, which can help reduce blistering. This healing gel also contains vitamins C and E as well as zinc, all of which are nutrients that speed burn healing. Research demonstrates that fresh aloe gel reduces inflammation and appears to enhance skin repair when applied to burns.

Pat yourself with black tea. To subdue sunburn pain as soon as it starts, rely on the tannic acid in tea. Make a cup of regular black or orange pekoe tea, and let it cool. Then pat it on your sunburned skin. You can use your fingertips or soak a cotton ball in the tea and apply. The tea's tannic acid helps restore the natural acid balance of your skin, which helps protect against infection. These tannins also activate proteins in the top layers of your skin to form a protective covering and help remove the feeling of heat. Reapply this tea as needed.

Soak in apple-cider vinegar. If your sunburn covers your body, fight the heat and pain by bathing in apple-cider vinegar. To prepare the bath, add a cup of apple-cider vinegar to a tub full of cool water. Relax, soak, and allow the astringent properties of the apple-cider vinegar to ease your pain.

Toothaches

Toothaches are like the class bully back in grammar school—impossible to ignore. You can try bypassing a painful tooth by chewing with the other teeth, but one false chew and *ouch!* the injured tooth delivers a jolt of pain.

Teeth ache because bacteria-laden plaque invades beneath the gum line, eventually irritating oh-so-sensitive nerve endings. Beyond pain, this plaque assault can leave behind cavities, tooth decay, or an abscess. So heed the pain warnings and see your dentist, pronto. Until you can get to her, try one of these herbal pain relievers to help you through the rough spots.

Stop pain with a dab of clove. To temporarily quell throbbing tooth pain, rub a drop of oil of clove directly on the aching tooth. If you don't have this oil handy, reach for a whole clove from your spice rack and rub the pointed end on the teeth closest to the aching area. Oil of clove

THE HERBAL KITCHEN
Peppermint Toothpaste

When she was a child, herbalist Rosemary Gladstar made regular trips to the dentist to have cavities treated. By the time she reached early adulthood, she needed root canal work. Fortunately, she found a way to bring her dental problems under control.

"About 15 years ago, I started making my own herbal toothpaste, and it has really cut down on my dental problems. Its alkalizing effect seems to reduce infections in my mouth," says Gladstar, who is director of the Sage Mountain Herbal Education Center in East Barre, Vermont, and author of *Herbal Healing for Women*.

She shares her recipe for a winning smile and great teeth.

- ¼ cup fine facial clay (available in health food stores)
- ¼ cup baking soda
- 1 teaspoon salt
- 1–2 drops peppermint essential oil
- ¼ teaspoon goldenseal (organically cultivated powder form)
- 1 teaspoon myrrh fine powder

Stir the clay, baking soda, salt, peppermint essential oil, goldenseal, and myrrh together in a bowl until they form a paste. Apply a dab of the paste to your wet toothbrush, then brush as usual. Rinse. Your herbal toothpaste will keep, so store it in a closed, decorative glass container on your bathroom sink. Gladstar says the peppermint provides a mouth-freshening flavor while the goldenseal and myrrh fight infection and receding gums.

contains 60 to 90 percent eugenol, a potent pain-deadening antimicrobial. Clove has earned the official endorsement of the Food and Drug Administration as an effective stopgap measure for tooth pain.

Compress pain with ginger. Diminish deep toothache pain by making a compress with ginger. This hot spice acts as a counterirritant, effectively distracting you from toothache pain. To make a compress for your aching tooth, mix a little powdered ginger in enough water to create a gooey paste. Dip a small cotton ball in the paste, then apply it directly to the tooth, trying to not get the paste on the gum. If you don't have ginger available, use cayenne pepper, following the same instructions. Cayenne contains salicylates, aspirin-like pain-subsiding chemicals.

Rely on this Chinese folk remedy. Since the fourth century, the Chinese have been reaching for sesame seeds to subdue tooth pain. Herbalists say sesame contains at least seven pain-relieving compounds. For best results, boil one part sesame seed with two parts water until half the liquid remains. Cool the resulting decoction and apply it directly to your aching tooth.

Munch willow bark. For short-term relief from toothaches, chew on a small wad of willow bark. Willow bark contains salicin, a chemical cousin of aspirin that shares its pain-relieving powers. You can also drink a tea made from this herb or take a tincture, following the label directions, to banish the ache.

Ulcers

Medical experts used to blame ulcers on stress, smoking, drinking excess alcohol, and eating rich or spicy foods. While any of these factors can cause ulcer pain, the scientific community has now found another, more common cause: a spiral-shaped bacterium answering to the name of *Helicobacter pylori.*

These airborne bacteria are still something of a mystery. Researchers aren't certain where they come from or how infection occurs. But they do know that they settle in the stomach or top part of the small intestine, where they penetrate the digestive tract's protective lining.

Whether your ulcer is the result of a bacterial invasion, stress, or lifestyle habits, the consequences are the same. Acid eats away at your stomach or intestinal lining, leaving a painful sore. Women with ulcers often experience a gnawing or burning pain in their abdomens, usually between meals or first thing in the morning. Some also vomit, lose weight, lose their appetites, develop blood in their stools, and feel nauseated.

It's important to see your doctor first for ulcer treatment. You can be tested for the presence of *Helicobacter pylori* and given medication to get rid of it. If that isn't the cause, or if you want to give your body extra help getting over a bout of painful ulcers, herbalists recommend these remedies that hasten healing and lessen the likelihood of repeat episodes.

Chew some licorice. To reduce the chances of recurring ulcers, take a natural product called deglycyrrhizinated licorice (DGL). Before or between meals slowly chew two tablets of DGL extract or swallow one-half teaspoon of the powder form. Stay on this herbal remedy for as long as symptoms persist. This herb contains several anti-ulcer compounds that protect the lining of the stomach and small intestine.

Sip anti-ulcer tea. Turn the volume down on ulcer pain, natural healers say, by drinking up to two cups of this herbal tea every day until your condition improves. Blend one teaspoon each of the dried herbs licorice root, marshmallow root, and chamomile flowers with one-half teaspoon each of Oregon grape root, hops, echinacea, and cinnamon in a pan with one quart of water. Bring to a boil, then simmer for 15 minutes. Remove from the heat and steep for 10 minutes. Strain the herbs and store the tea in the refrigerator until you're ready to drink it.

These herbs work in tandem to lower stomach acid levels, and they decrease the chances of a repeat ulcer attack.

Enjoy a fruit-and-spice drink. You can soothe a sore stomach by sipping a fruity anti-ulcer beverage between meals. Put blueberries and a banana in a blender. Add ground cinnamon, ground cloves, and ground ginger to taste. Blend until smooth and garnish each serving with a peppermint sprig. The tasty, no-fat ingredients in this recipe all contain significant amounts of stomach-soothing, ulcer-fighting compounds.

SLIPPERY ELM
Good for: irritation and inflammation of the reproductive, digestive, and respiratory systems as well as of the urinary tract

Urinary Tract Infections

When you gotta go, you gotta go. But if you have a frequent, urgent need to urinate accompanied by a burning sensation or a pain in your urethra, you may have a urinary tract infection (UTI).

Urinary tract infections occur when bacteria invade the urethra, the little pipe through which your urine exits. Less-than-sanitary toilet habits contribute to getting UTIs. So do using diaphragms and spermicides as well as douches or feminine deodorants. Peak times for these infections generally are just before menstruation, following intercourse, and at menopause when the vaginal walls are more susceptible to bacteria, say women doctors.

One out of every five women will get a UTI sometime in her life—eight times more frequently than their male counterparts. And once you have one infection, your chances for more infections rise. You can lower your chances of a future UTI attack by practicing good hygiene, such as wiping from front to back after you use the toilet. This keeps bacteria away from the urethra. Drink up to eight glasses of water per day and urinate as needed. Holding back only allows bacteria to grow.

See your doctor if you see blood in your urine, which is an indication that you may have a more serious bladder or kidney condition. Most likely, your doctor will give you antibiotics to kill the bacterial invaders that caused the infection.

If you're otherwise healthy, UTIs usually clear themselves within three to seven days. But most women don't want to endure the pain that long. Turn to these herbal helpers that outwit the bacteria and fortify the mucous membranes that line the urinary tract against infection. Since prolonged urinary tract infections can damage your kidneys, it is important to see a doctor if it doesn't clear after seven days.

Drink plenty of cranberry juice. To prevent bacteria from sticking to bladder walls, herbalists suggest drinking up to 17 ounces of cranberry juice per day. Scientific studies show that this fruit contains arbutin, a chemical compound that acts as both an antibiotic and a diuretic.

Try an antiseptic formula. Fight infection and soothe urination pain with uva-ursi, corn silk, and echinacea. Herbalists recommend taking 10 drops of each herb in tincture form in one-half cup of water or a noncitrus juice, as needed. Drink this natural antiseptic to kill bacteria in your urinary tract. Just don't use uva-ursi for more than two weeks without the supervision of a qualified herbalist. Also, don't use it if you have kidney disease, because it contains tannins that can cause further kidney damage. Tannins can also irritate your stomach.

Bathe in relief. To relieve the external burning of a UTI and hasten healing, sit in a bath that's half-filled with warm water and a few drops of essential oils, natural healers recommend. In a small dish, combine three drops of sandalwood essential oil, two drops of tea tree essential oil, one drop of chamomile essential oil, and two tablespoons of honey. Pour two tablespoons of apple-cider vinegar, which is a mild astringent, into the bath and then add the honey mixture, which helps hold the oils together and keeps them from floating on top of the water. Soak for 20 minutes.

Sandalwood is antibacterial, tea tree is antiseptic, and chamomile is anti-inflammatory.

Vaginal Dryness

Sex should feel wonderful. But intercourse can be downright painful if your vagina isn't well-lubricated, a condition that may be temporary or, if a result of natural hormonal changes, long-lasting.

After menopause, your vaginal lining thins and dries because of dwindling supplies of the female hormone estrogen. Estrogen helps keep vaginal tissue moist and healthy. In addition, menopause causes your vagina to shrink and lose muscle tone.

While vaginal dryness poses no serious threat to your health, it does make sex uncomfortable—and sometimes, impossible. Here are some lubricating herbal solutions to help keep your love life flowing.

WOMAN TO WOMAN
She Got Rid of a Kidney Infection

Even after consulting with three doctors, Linda Copeland, a 42-year-old hairdresser and mother of three from Gresham, Oregon, couldn't get relief from persistent kidney pains that lingered after she had managed to clear up a urinary tract infection. It took a naturopathic physician at her church picnic to get her the relief she needed. Here's her story.

I had a urinary tract infection last winter, so I went to my family doctor, who gave me antibiotics. The antibiotics got rid of the infection, but not the pain in my kidneys.

The aching, burning pain lingered for months. It got worse whenever I ate acidic or spicy foods—even melons, strawberries, and spaghetti sauce. I started on a bland diet in the hope of finding some relief, but I was afraid that something was wrong with my kidneys, so I went to a urologist and then to a gastroenterologist. They told me that the antibiotics had cleared up the infection and that there should be no reason for my kidneys to hurt. But I knew my body. Something was wrong.

By the time I saw Dr. Jennifer Reid at our church barbecue, I was at my wit's end. I first met Jennifer in a Bible study class back when she was going to school to study

Try this aloe-powered liquid lube. Keep your vagina well-lubricated with this herbal "moisturizer," suggest natural healers. Blend equal parts of distilled witch hazel and pure aloe vera gel. For added slickness, mix in some slippery elm powder, say herbalists. Use as needed before and during sex.

Apply rejuvenation oil. Moisturize your vagina with an herbalist-recommended vaginal rejuvenation oil blend. Combine two ounces of almond oil or vegetable oil, six drops each of rose geranium and lavender essential oils, and 1,500 international units (IU) of vitamin E oil. (You naturopathic medicine. We became friends. The day of the barbecue, we started talking. She suggested I come to her office that week. We bartered. I offered to cut her husband's hair in exchange for her advice.

She took my medical history, examined me, and then suggested that I take slippery elm. I had never tried herbs before, but I trusted Jennifer. I looked up this herb in a nutritional healing book, which talked about its cleansing effects on the kidneys and colon. I thought of it as a natural Pepto-Bismol for my kidneys. I took some capsules every day, usually with a warm cup of herbal tea. Within a couple of days, I felt better. Within a week, the pain was totally gone.

Now I try to avoid antibiotics whenever possible. Instead, I take cranberry tablets and the slippery elm capsules from the health food store. Somehow, the slippery elm seems to coat everything, so that even drinking something as acidic as orange juice no longer causes my kidneys to hurt.

I was also diagnosed with interstitial cystitis (inflammation of the bladder), and slippery elm helped to decrease my urgency to urinate. I found myself making far fewer trips to the bathroom.

Since Jennifer introduced me to this herb, I feel like I've discovered a whole new world of options. If my family doctor or conventional medicine can't help me, I know I can always try herbal remedies.

can use the oil from vitamin E capsules.) Apply this oil blend inside the vagina as needed to restore moisture.

Vaginal Itch

Equally uncomfortable and embarrassing, few things are as maddening as vaginal itching. After all, how is a lady to find relief?

Itching may be a sign that you may have a yeast infection, bacterial infection, or even a sexually transmitted disease such as chlamydia, herpes, or gonorrhea. Or the delicate skin in and around your vagina may be reacting to chemicals in douches, bubble baths, or soaps. Changes in hormone levels, especially before menstruation, during pregnancy, and after menopause, can also cause that itchy feeling.

Medical experts advise against treating a vaginal itch on your own unless you know exactly what you're dealing with. Check with a doctor to pinpoint the cause. Often, she will prescribe antibiotics or vaginal creams to prevent complications and soothe the irritation quickly. After you've seen your doctor and have your medical prescriptions, try these botanically based helpers to assist in relieving itching and discomfort.

Stop the itch with Caladium. Reach for relief with homeopathic Caladium, a remedy herbalists highly recommend. Take a 6X dose up to three times a day for no longer than three days. But if it is not helping after three doses, discontinue use because it's probably not the right remedy for your condition. The notation 6X is a standard measurement in homeopathy and refers to a remedy's potency, which is listed on the label.

Soak in apple-cider vinegar. To banish many types of vaginitis, add three cups of apple-cider vinegar to a hot bath. Soak in the tub for at least 20 minutes, spreading your legs to allow the water to flow around your vagina. Herbalists say vinegar baths help restore normal vaginal acidity.

Varicose Veins

The veins in your legs are among the longest in your body. When they're working properly, a series of 10 to 20 tiny valves inside them acts like locks in a canal, allowing blood returning to the heart to collect at various points and then move on its way.

But sometimes, good veins go bad. Valves weaken, allowing blood that was headed up to your heart to trickle back down and pool instead. As a result, sections of your veins swell.

The word *varicose* means swollen. Because they're so extremely dilated, varicose veins seem to nearly pop from the skin. They're most noticeable in the legs, since standing upright exerts tremendous pressure on the blood vessels down there. Women are four times more prone to varicose veins than men are, perhaps because pregnancy increases pressure on the veins in the legs. Obesity, aging, and standing for hours on the job also cause vein swelling.

In most instances, varicose veins can make your legs feel tired, tight, and heavy. In rare cases, this condition can lead to a blood clot. If you experience sudden, painful swelling of one leg with tenderness in the calf muscle, seek medical help right away. A blood clot may have formed in one of the deep veins of the leg.

If you have garden-variety varicose veins, or if you want to avoid developing them in the first place, these herbs can help keep your blood vessels strong and elastic, improve circulation, and make those purple bulges less unsightly.

Choose bilberry for stronger veins. If you want to improve the appearance of varicosity and strengthen your leg veins, take 80 milligrams of bilberry in capsule form three times a day—at breakfast, lunch, and again at dinner. Bilberry restores the connective tissue sheath surrounding veins. This prevents the veins from bulging, so excess blood won't start to collect. In addition, bilberry also helps circulation by stimulating new capillary formation and strengthening capillary walls.

Ease the bulge with an herbal formula. Prevent existing varicose veins from getting any worse with this herbalist-recommended recipe. Combine two parts ginkgo tincture, one part ginger tincture, and one part cinnamon tincture. Take 30 drops of this combination, mixed with a liquid (such as tea, juice, or water), three times per day.

After a month, re-evaluate your condition. You may or may not need to use the formula a little longer. Cinnamon is an herb that increases circulation. Ginkgo is a highly regarded treatment for a variety of blood vessel disorders. Ginger aids the cardiovascular system. It may make your gallbladder secrete more bile, however; so if you have gallstones, don't use therapeutic amounts of dried gingerroot or powder without guidance from a health care practitioner.

Go with a premade vein toner. A compound in horse chestnut helps to strengthen the capillary cells and reduce fluid leakage. Strengthening capillary tone can improve the appearance of varicose veins.

Horse chestnut is best used as a minor ingredient in an overall formula that includes other herbs. Look for commercial formulas of liquid tinctures or capsules that contain some horse chestnut—often, they are available by mail order.

Vomiting

Yes, it's unpleasant. But vomiting is often the most effective way for your body to eject

SPEARMINT
Good for: indigestion during pregnancy and combating midafternoon slumps

harmful substances—from tainted food to too much alcohol. More often than not, you're better off letting it all out than suppressing a retch.

Fortunately, one good upchuck is usually all it takes to relieve most nausea. But afterward, you may feel dehydrated, drained, and achy. Or you may be plagued by the dreaded dry heaves. That's when the herbal remedies listed below can help most.

If your vomiting goes on and on, however, check with your doctor. She should check that you don't have a serious condition like toxicity, an infection of the digestive tract, or parasites.

Find relief in the spice rack. If the flu or tainted food causes repeat-performance vomiting as well as diarrhea, sip a tea made of cinnamon and ginger, herbalists suggest. Mix one teaspoon of dried cinnamon with one-half teaspoon of grated fresh ginger and add them to a cup of boiling water. Steep for 10 to 15 minutes, then strain and sip. Cinnamon is a natural astringent that dries up loose stools. Herbalists regard ginger as the premier herb for vomiting and nausea.

Calm with peppermint. A cup of peppermint tea can curb the muscle spasms in the digestive tract that often accompany vomiting. Mix a tablespoon of fresh peppermint leaves or a teaspoon of dried ones into a cup of hot water. Cover for five minutes to keep the healing volatile oils from escaping. Then strain and drink.

Soak up relief with an herbal bath. If nausea leads to vomiting, you might throw up any remedies you've swallowed. If that's the case, then try a soothing herb soak instead. Mix a tablespoon of fresh ginger or any amount, from a teaspoon to a tablespoon, of powdered ginger with a quart of just-boiled water. Let the water cool so you don't scald yourself, then soak your hands or feet until the vomiting subsides.

Warts

Usually painless, warts are nevertheless far from flattering. These knobby little skin lesions most commonly appear on the hands, fingers, forearms, knees, face, and feet.

Warts, which are actually benign skin tumors, are caused by a family of viruses called human papillomavirus (HPV). A suppressed immune system seems to increase a woman's susceptibility to them.

Getting rid of warts doesn't always eliminate the virus that caused them in the first place, so natural healers suggest a two-pronged strategy for achieving a lasting solution: Bolster your immune system so that it can better battle viruses and use herbs that work on the surface to shrink these little growths.

Bite back with birch bark. Make warts disappear safely and naturally with birch bark. People all over the world have relied on this herb for centuries. If you have access to fresh birch bark, tape a piece of moistened bark, with the inner side down, directly to the wart. If you can't get your hands on some bark, brew some birch bark tea by adding a teaspoon or two of powdered bark to a cup of boiling water. Steep for 10 minutes. You can drink it as a tea or rub it directly on the wart.

Birch bark contains two antiviral compounds, betulin and betulinic acid, in addition to salicylates, which are approved by the Food and Drug Administration to treat warts.

Fight the virus with echinacea. Fortify your immune system so that it can defeat wart viruses by taking two 250-milligram capsules of echinacea twice per day, natural healers recommend. Echinacea boosts immune-system functioning.

Bombard with basil. Counter the HPV virus with crushed, fresh basil leaves. Simply pack the crushed leaves over the wart and cover with a bandage. Apply fresh basil daily for five to seven days. This aromatic herb contains many antiviral compounds that have the potential to make warts disappear.

Water Retention

Swollen feet? Bloated abdomen? Fingers so puffy your rings get stuck? Most times, you can blame that bloated feeling on a lower level of the female hormone progesterone. This decline usually occurs about a week to 10 days before your menstrual period begins.

As progesterone levels fall, your salt levels rise, so you retain water. The more salt you stock, the more water is retained throughout your body. Strange as it may sound, herbalists and conventional medical practitioners agree that you must actually drink *more* water to deflate water retention. At the same time, cut back on your salt intake. These front-line defenses help dilute sodium and assist your kidneys in flushing it out of your body.

Before trying herbal treatments, consult your doctor to find out exactly what's causing your water retention. Sometimes it's a symptom of a serious heart or kidney problem. If you have a condition called pitting edema, in which you've retained so much water that

---

WART BE GONE!

With just a drop or two a day of an easy-to-prepare recipe, you can make warts disappear.

The essential oils of tea tree and thuja both possess antiviral and antifungal properties, making them powerful agents against warts, says Gail Ulrich, an herbalist, director of the Blazing Star Herbal School in Shelburne Falls, Massachusetts, and author of *Herbs to Boost Immunity*. Combined with a few other products, they make for a wonderful wart-dissolving oil.

You'll use only a little bit each day, so the solution should last for about two to three weeks. By then, the wart should be gone. You'll need castor oil, thuja essential oil, tea tree essential oil, and vitamin E capsules.

---

pressing on a swollen spot leaves indentations on your skin, or if you retain water during pregnancy, it's also very important to contact your doctor.

If, on the other hand, you have a simple but irritating case of water retention, turn to the

In a small wide-mouth bottle or jar with a lid, combine one tablespoon of castor oil, 25 drops (or about one-quarter teaspoon) of thuja essential oil, and 25 drops (or about one-quarter teaspoon) of tea tree essential oil. Using small scissors or a needle, snip or puncture two vitamin E capsules (each containing 400 international units). Squeeze out the vitamin E oil. Mix all the ingredients well.

Because the oil may burn the skin, cover the area surrounding the wart with a salve, such as vitamin E oil or lanolin. Using a cotton-tipped swab, a toothpick, or a dropper, apply the mixture to the wart. Place a bandage over the wart. Reapply the solution once a day until the wart disappears. Keep the solution in a covered bottle or jar, which you should store in a cool, dark place.

herbal pharmacy for gentle diuretics that help flush excess fluids from your body.

Diminish bloating with corn. If you're looking for a safe, effective diuretic, herbalists suggest corn silk tea. Steep one tablespoon of dried corn silk in a cup of just-boiled water for five minutes. Drink up to three cups per day, but avoid this herb at night—otherwise, you will be interrupting your sleep with trips to the bathroom.

Corn silk, those fine, threadlike strands jutting from the top of an ear of corn, prompts the kidneys to flush out excess water. Researchers aren't certain which compounds account for this fluid-flushing quality, but they know it works. Instead of sipping this tea, you could also use several cups of it as the flavorful base for vegetable soup. Don't use silk from store-bought corn for this tea, unless you know that it has been organically grown without pesticides. Otherwise, purchase corn silk in a health food store or by mail order from companies that sell organic herbs.

Drain with dandelion. Encourage more frequent urination, which eliminates extra fluid, by quaffing dandelion leaf tea, herbal healers say. Add one cup boiling water to one teaspoon dried dandelion leaf. Let it steep for five minutes before straining. Drink up to three cups per day for a few days before your monthly period is to start. If you are on medication, check with your doctor to make sure your medication is not a diuretic (something that causes fluid loss), as are certain blood pressure medications. If so, avoid dandelion.

Try an herbal combo. For variety, natural healers suggest this diuretic tea, which taps the effectiveness of both dandelion and corn silk as well as other diuretic herbs. Combine the following dried herbs: two teaspoons dandelion root and one-half teaspoon each of nettle leaf, oatstraw, fennel seed, and corn silk. Add the herbs to a pot of boiling water. Cover, turn off the heat, and steep for 20 minutes. Strain, and drink one to two cups per day as needed.

Wound Healing

You nicked your hand while pruning the hedge, and weeks later, it still hasn't healed completely. The scrape you got from a bicycle spill on gravel refuses to disappear. So does that little incision on your arm, where the doctor removed a suspicious-looking mole.

In ideal conditions, a cut, scrape, or surgical incision mends swiftly and neatly. No sign of infection. No long-lasting red mark. No need to wear bandages for weeks on end. But conditions are often not so ideal. Everything from dirt and microbes to poor circulation can slow the healing process. Diabetes or hardening of the arteries— medical conditions that cause poor circulation— can also prevent wounds from healing. Don't try to self-treat a wound that won't mend, particularly if you have one of these conditions. See a doctor.

Otherwise, for a minor, nonthreatening wound, botanical remedies might help. Before using one, wash the injured site thoroughly with mild soap and water. Then enhance healing with these tissue-mending herbs.

Draw out debris with astringent herbs. If infection or small pieces of dirt slow healing, herbalists recommend an herbal soak. For wounds that you can easily immerse in a basin or large bowl, make a strong tea using one quart of water and one-half cup of either wild geranium, dried oak bark, or dried witch hazel. Simmer the tea for about 30 minutes, then strain. Soak the wound in the comfortably hot tea for at least 15 minutes to draw out debris and infection.

If the wound can't be soaked easily, use the strong tea mixture to make a compress. Soak a clean cloth in the tea, but don't wring it out. Lay the wet cloth over the wound. Every few minutes, rinse the cloth in the tea and reapply.

These astringent herbs have been used traditionally to clean wounds and make torn skin pull together. Combined with warm water, these herbs act like vacuum cleaners, sucking out debris.

Hasten healing with calendula. Once the wound is clean and infection-free, speed healing and lessen scarring with a calendula compress, herbalists suggest. Pour a cup of boiling water over one teaspoon of dried calendula petals and steep for 10 minutes. Then soak a clean cloth in the liquid and apply the cloth to the wound. Or, you can buy commercial skin creams that contain calendula from health food stores. German medicinal herb experts endorse this herb to hasten skin healing.

Rely on echinacea. To fend off inflammation in hard-to-heal wounds, herbalists recommend a compress made with echinacea. Mix one part echinacea tincture with three parts water and apply to the wound with a clean cloth. Leave this compress in place for 10 to 15 minutes. Reapply four times per day until the wound is clearly healing.

YARROW
Good for: a poultice for bleeding and wound healing

Wrinkles

Wrinkles are a small price to pay for smiling at the skies as you watch hawks soar. Or laughing at a good joke. Or snuggling up to a big, fluffy pillow as you sleep.

In fact, if you've lived at all, you probably have wrinkles. The crinkles and creases usually start to surface after age 30 as collagen and elastin (protein fibers that give skin support and elasticity) start to break down.

Unprotected sun exposure is the most frequent cause of wrinkles; more than 90 percent of premature aging is a direct result of the sun's ultraviolet rays. The sun wreaks havoc on the skin by breaking down collagen and elastin, causing your skin to lose tone. Smoking also ages your skin prematurely by constricting blood vessels and impairing circulation to the skin.

It's difficult to avoid or erase wrinkles completely, but there are plenty of lifestyle and herbal options that can minimize them. Drink plenty of water (at least eight eight-ounce glasses per day), don't smoke, wear sunscreen daily, avoid tanning salons, exercise regularly, and include some healthy fats in your diet, such as olive or canola oil. These lifestyle adjustments will give a glow and supple feeling to your skin. So can the following herbal wrinkle warriors.

Tame deep wrinkles with a botanical face treatment. For pronounced wrinkles, use a strong botanical remedy made with lemon and water. Herbal treatments can remove the upper layers of dead skin and, over time, can minimize wrinkles by encouraging the growth of new skin, say women herbalists. Before you apply this treatment, clean your skin with a non-oily cleanser. Make sure your hands are clean, too.

Mix equal parts of lemon juice and distilled water. Use your fingers to pat the mixture on your face, being careful not to get any in your eyes or on your lips. Your face should feel a little puckery, and it may sting slightly. Leave the treatment on for five minutes, then rinse with

> ### AN APPLE A DAY TAKES WRINKLES AWAY
>
> Want a 25-cent alternative to the $75 bottles of alpha hydroxy acid cream women are buying to smooth out their wrinkles? Then go to the grocery store and buy an apple.
>
> Alpha hydroxy acids, which peel away layers of dead skin and expose the new skin underneath for a smoother appearance, naturally occur in fruits such as apples. Try using a homemade apple face mask to improve the condition of your skin, suggests Jenny McFeely, a member of Britain's National Institute of Medical Herbalists and a professional member of the American Herbalists Guild, who is from Scottsdale, Arizona.
>
> Before making an apple face mask, clean your skin with a non-oily cleanser. Then cut up an apple and place it in a blender. Puree the apple until it is moist and pulpy. Smear it all over your face, and leave it there for 15 to 20 minutes.
>
> Use this treatment three times a week, and you'll soon get the same results you would expect from that expensive lotion that comes in a fancy bottle.

lukewarm water and apply a nonpetroleum moisturizer. Use a peel three times a week, and small wrinkles may completely diminish within three months.

Concoct a natural face-lift. Tighten wrinkles temporarily with an egg facial, which will keep skin smooth-looking for up to five hours. If you have oily skin, use only the egg whites. For normal or dry skin, use one whole egg. Whip the egg with one teaspoon of dried or fresh lavender flowers and apply to your clean face. Leave on until the egg hardens. Lay a wet washcloth (use tepid water) on your face to soften the egg. Then glide the egg off with the washcloth. Finish with a toner and a nonpetroleum moisturizer. This remedy works great before going out to a special event where you want to look especially nice.

Safe Use of Herbs in This Book

While herbs are generally safe and cause few, if any, side effects, researchers and specialists in natural medicine caution that you should use them responsibly. Foremost, if you are under a doctor's care for any health condition or are taking any medication, don't take any herb without your doctor knowing about it. Certain natural substances can change the way your body absorbs and processes certain medications. Also, if you are pregnant, do not self-treat yourself with any natural remedy without the consent of your obstetrician or midwife. The same goes for nursing mothers and women trying to conceive.

Below are cautions and guides for the herbs mentioned in this book that can potentially cause adverse reactions in some people. Though such occurrences are rare, you should be aware of what they are and discontinue use of the herb if you experience an unusual reaction. Also, do not exceed the recommended dosages—more is *not* better.

By familiarizing yourself with this list, you can enjoy the world of natural healing and use this book with confidence.

Herb	Safe Use Guidelines and Possible Side Effects
Aloe	Do not use gel externally on any surgical incision, because it may delay wound healing.
Angelica	Use sparingly and only for short periods of time. Increases sun sensitivity and may cause skin rash, so avoid prolonged sun exposure.
Arnica	Do not use on broken skin.
Basil	Do not take large amounts (several cups a day) for extended periods.
Bearberry	Do not use for more than two weeks without the supervision of a qualified herbalist. Do not use if you have kidney disease, because it contains tannins, which can cause further kidney damage. Tannins can also irritate the stomach.
Birch	Do not take if you need to avoid aspirin, since its active ingredient, salicin, is related to aspirin.
Black cohosh	Do not use for more than six months.
Black haw	If you have a history of kidney stones, do not take without medical supervision, because it contains oxalates, which can cause kidney stones.
Bladderwrack	May reduce absorption of iron, sodium, and potassium, so do not take for more than six weeks. Not recommended if you have hyperthyroidism. Can aggravate existing acne.
Bloodroot	May cause nausea and vomiting in doses higher than 5 to 10 drops of tincture twice a day. Safe when used in commercial dental products.
Cayenne	May irritate the gastrointestinal tract if taken on an empty stomach. Don't use near eyes.

Herb	Safe Use Guidelines and Possible Side Effects
Chamomile	May trigger an allergic reaction in people allergic to closely related plants such as ragweed, asters, and chrysanthemums.
Chasteberry	May counter the effectiveness of birth control pills.
Coleus forskohlii	May enhance the effects of medications for asthma or high blood pressure with negative results, so do not use unless under medical supervision.
Coltsfoot	Do not use for more than one week unless under supervised care by a doctor or qualified herbalist.
Comfrey	For external use only. Do not use on deep or infected wounds, because it can promote surface healing too quickly and not allow healing of underlying tissue.
Dandelion root	If you have gallbladder disease, do not use dandelion preparations without medical approval.
Dong quai	Do not use while menstruating, spotting, or bleeding heavily, since it can increase blood loss.
Echinacea	Do not use if you're allergic to closely related plants such as ragweed, asters, and chrysanthemums. Do not use if you have tuberculosis or an autoimmune condition such as lupus or multiple sclerosis, because echinacea stimulates the immune system.
Ephedra	Do not use without the supervision of a medical doctor.
Eucalyptus	Do not use if you have inflammatory disease of the bile ducts or gastrointestinal tract or severe liver disease. May cause nausea, vomiting, and diarrhea in doses higher than four grams a day.
Fennel	Do not use medicinally for more than six weeks without supervision by a qualified herbalist.
Feverfew	If chewed, fresh leaves can cause mouth sores in some people.
Flax	Take with at least eight ounces of water.
Garlic	Do not use supplements if you are on anticoagulants or about to undergo surgery, because garlic thins the blood and may increase bleeding. Do not use if you're taking hypoglycemic drugs.
Gentian	May cause nausea and vomiting in large doses. Do not use if you have high blood pressure, ulcers, or gastrointestinal irritation and inflammation.
Ginger	Dried root or powder used in therapeutic amounts may increase bile secretions in people with gallstones. Fresh ginger is safe when used as a spice.
Ginkgo	Do not use if you are taking antidepressant MAO inhibitor drugs, aspirin or other nonsteroidal anti-inflammatory medications, or blood-thinning medications. In doses higher than 240 milligrams of concentrated extract, it can cause rash, diarrhea, and vomiting.
Ginseng	May cause irritability if taken with caffeine or other stimulants. Do not take if you have high blood pressure.
Goldenrod	Do not use if you have a chronic kidney disorder.
Goldenseal	Do not use if you have high blood pressure.

Herb	Safe Use Guidelines and Possible Side Effects
Hawthorn	If you have a cardiovascular condition, do not take hawthorn regularly for more than a few weeks without medical supervision. You may require lower doses of other medications, such as drugs for high blood pressure. If you have low blood pressure caused by heart valve problems, do not use without medical supervision.
Hops	Do not take if you are prone to depression.
Horse chestnut	Can interfere with the action of other drugs, especially blood thinners. Can irritate the gastrointestinal tract.
Horsetail	Do not use the tincture if you have heart or kidney problems. May cause a thiamin deficiency. Do not take more than two grams per day of powdered extract or take for prolonged periods.
Jamaican dogwood	Do not exceed the recommended dose and use only as needed.
Kava kava	Do not take with alcohol or barbiturates. Do not take more than the recommended dose on package. Use caution when driving or operating equipment, since this herb causes drowsiness.
Licorice	Do not use if you have diabetes, high blood pressure, liver or kidney disorders, or low potassium levels. Do not use daily for more than four to six weeks because overuse can lead to water retention, high blood pressure caused by potassium loss, or impaired heart and kidney function.
Marshmallow	May slow the absorption of medications taken at the same time.
Meadowsweet	Do not use if you need to avoid aspirin, since its active ingredient is related to aspirin.
Myrrh	Can cause diarrhea and irritation of the kidneys. Do not use if you have uterine bleeding for any reason.
Nettle	If you have allergies, your symptoms may worsen, so take only once a day for the first few days.
Oak	Do not use externally on extensively damaged skin.
Oatstraw	Do not use if you have celiac disease (gluten intolerance), because it contains gluten, a grain protein.
Psyllium	Take one hour after other drugs. Take with at least eight ounces of water.
Rosemary	May cause excessive menstrual bleeding.
Rue	Can irritate the gastrointestinal tract and should not be used by individuals with poor kidney function. Can cause sensitivity to the sun.
Sage	In therapeutic amounts, it can increase the sedative side effects of drugs. Do not use if you have hypoglycemia or are undergoing anticonvulsant therapy. Safe when used as a spice.
St. John's wort	Can cause sensitivity to the sun. Do not use with antidepressants without medical approval.
Sarsaparilla	May speed elimination of prescription medications, thereby requiring an increase in their dose in order to be effective.

Herb	Safe Use Guidelines and Possible Side Effects
Sassafras	Long-term use of sassafras tea is not recommended. Do not take more than the recommended dose.
Shepherd's purse	Do not use if you have a history of kidney stones.
Tea	Fermented black tea is not recommended for excessive or long-term use because it is a nervous system stimulant. Women with irregular heartbeats should limit their intake of green tea to no more than two cups daily because the caffeine and other alkaloids can speed up heart rates. Its bitter taste stimulates gastric acid production, so it should be consumed in limited amounts by people with stomach ulcers.
Turmeric	Do not use therapeutically if you have high stomach acid or ulcers, gallstones, or bile duct obstruction. Safe for use as a spice.
Valerian	Do not use with sleep-enhancing or mood-regulating medications, because it may intensify their effects. May cause heart palpitations and nervousness in sensitive individuals. If such stimulant action occurs, discontinue use.
Wild cherry	For occasional use only. Don't exceed recommended dose.
Willow	Because of similar active ingredients, follow the same cautions with willow as you would for aspirin.
Yellow dock	If you have a history of kidney stones, do not take without medical supervision, since it contains oxalates and tannins that may adversely affect this condition.

Safe Use of Essential Oils in This Book

Essential oils are inhaled or placed on the skin, but they should never be taken internally because they're so concentrated that they can be toxic. One exception is peppermint oil, which can be ingested in capsule form. If you have gallbladder or liver disease, however, you shouldn't do so without a doctor's consent. Peppermint oil may also lead to stomach upset in sensitive individuals.

Never apply essential oils neat (undiluted) unless otherwise indicated. Dilute them first in a neutral base, which can be an oil (such as almond), cream, or gel. Many essential oils may cause skin irritation or allergic reactions in people with sensitive skin.

Before applying any new oil to your skin, always do a patch test. Put a few drops of diluted oil on the back of your wrist. Wait for an hour or more. If irritation or redness occur, bathe the area with cold water. In the future, prepare a dilution with half the amount of essential oil or avoid it altogether. As with herbs, do not use essential oils without first consulting your doctor if you are pregnant or nursing. Essential oils should be stored in dark bottles, away from light and heat, and out of the reach of children and pets.

Essential Oil	Safe Use Guidelines and Possible Side Effects
Angelica	Do not use topically if you have diabetes. When using the root oil, avoid direct sunlight because uneven skin coloring can occur.
Basil	May irritate the skin if used in a high concentration.
Bergamot	Avoid direct sunlight after topical application because uneven skin coloring can occur (except with the bergapten-free type).
Cedarwood	Use in moderation (no more than two weeks at a time). May irritate the skin if used in a high concentration. Atlas cedarwood is considered safe.
Clove	Use in moderation (no more than two weeks at a time). This oil is used undiluted as anesthesia in dentistry.
Eucalyptus	Use in moderation (no more than two weeks at a time). May irritate the skin if used in a high concentration. Do not apply externally to the face.
Garlic	May irritate the skin if used in a high concentration.
Juniper	Use in moderation (no more than two weeks at a time). Do not use if you have kidney disease.
Lavender	Can be used neat, but keep it away from your eyes.
Lemon	May irritate the skin if used in a high concentration. Avoid direct sunlight after topical application because uneven skin coloring can occur.
Lemongrass	For topical use only. Do not inhale.
Orange	Avoid direct sunlight after topical application because uneven skin coloring can occur.
Peppermint	May irritate the skin if used in a high concentration. Do not use on your face.

Essential Oil	Safe Use Guidelines and Possible Side Effects
Rosemary	Do not use if you have hypertension. Because of its powerful action on the nervous system, do not use if you have epilepsy.
Sage	Spanish sage can be used in moderation (no more than two weeks at a time), but do not use it at all if you have hypertension or epilepsy. Do not use clary sage with alcohol; this sage can cause a narcotic effect and exaggerate drunkenness. Do not use common sage at all.
Sandalwood	Can be used neat as a perfume, but keep it away from your eyes.
Tea tree	May be applied neat to the skin.
Thuja	Use cautiously. Not recommended for general use in massage oils, baths, or aromatherapy. May irritate the skin if used in a high concentration.
Thyme	Do not use red thyme. White and common thyme may irritate the skin if used in a high concentration and should not be used if you have hypertension.
Ylang-ylang	Can be used neat as a perfume, but keep it away from your eyes. Use in moderation since its strong smell can cause nausea or headaches.

Herb Index

Boldface page references indicate illustrations. Underscored references indicate boxed text.

A

Almond, 20, 153–54
Aloe, 2, 3, 4, 31–32, 31, 50, 69, 80, 84, 154, 154, 158, 167
Angelica, 32, 73, 118–19, 167, 171
Apple-cider vinegar, 95, 155, 159
Arnica, 3, 82, 135, 167
Asian ginseng, 43, 124, 126
Astragalus, 32–33, 32–33, 40, 77
Avocado, 142

B

Basil, 33, 40, 71, 105, 126, 162, 167, 171
Bay leaves, 98
Bearberry, 33–34, 81, 167
Bergamot, 171
Bilberry, 160
Birch bark, 161, 167
Black cohosh, 34, 66, 81, 111, 117, 127, 128, 139, 145, 167
Black haw, 34, 129, 167
Black tea, 113, 154–55, 170
Bladderwrack, 144, 167
Bloodroot, 95, 167
Blueberry, 99
Blue cohosh, 34
Bromelain, 135
Burdock, 34–35, 68–69, 75, 84, 94, 113–14
Butternut, 113

C

Caladium, 159
Calendula, 3, 14, 35, 77, 80, 82, 84, 86, 93–94, 101, 153–54, 164
Cardamom, 78
Cascara sagrada, 50
Castor oil, 86–87, 136
Cayenne, 65–66, 75, 123, 135, 143, 167
Cedarwood, 171

Chamomile

Chamomile, 3, 14, 18–19, 35–36, 59, 59, 61–62, 83, 92, 107, 111–12, 149–50, 158, 168
Chasteberry, 2, 12, 36, 66, 103, 119, 131, 139, 145–46, 168
Chickweed, 78–79, 117
Chinese skullcap, 53
Cinnamon, 78, 99, 160
Clove, 155, 171
Clover, red, 52
Cocoa, 92
Coconut oil, 92
Cohosh. See Black cohosh; Blue cohosh
Coleus forskohlii, 76, 115, 168
Coltsfoot, 50, 168
Comfrey, 8, 36, 62, 84, 94, 136, 168
Coneflower. See Echinacea
Corn silk, 157, 163
Cramp bark, 36–37, 110, 119, 129
Cranberry, 157

D

Damiana, 61, 97, 104
Dandelion root, 37, 37, 65, 69, 72, 75, 90, 97, 97, 119, 129, 132, 137, 144, 150, 163, 168
Deglycyrrhizinated licorice (DGL), 47, 111, 115, 156
Dill, 112
Dock root, 72
Dong quai, 38, 119, 168

E

Echinacea, 2, 3, 12, 38, 64, 67, 80, 85, 88, 98, 102, 107, 113–14, 124, 147, 150, 157, 161–62, 164, 168
Elderberry, 77, 88
Elderflowers, 70, 109
Elecampane, 92
Ephedra, 144, 168
Eucalyptus, 19, 39, 81–82, 87, 107, 151, 168, 171

Evening primrose, 38–39, 39–40, 76, 81, 100, 102
Eyebright, 70, 151

F

Fennel, 40, 80, 106, **113**, 119, 149, 168
Fen-phen, 144
Fenugreek, 116
Feverfew, 14, 40–41, 110, 132, 168
Flaxseed, 90, 100, 115, 168

G

Garlic, 2, 10, 40, 41–42, 41, 50, 70–71, 75, 86, 88, 102, 115, 115, 116, **119**, 125, 168, 171
Genistein, 103
Gentian, 118–19, 142, 168
Geranium, 130
Ginger, 42, 74, 75, 77, 88–90, 118, **121**, 132–33, 132, 137, 155–56, 160, 168
Gingerroot, 3
Ginkgo, 10, 10, 42, 43, 68, 70, 71, 76, 125–26, 134, 160, 168
Ginseng, 2, 43, 65, 66, 71, 98, 105, 109, 119, 121, 124, **125**, 126, 153, 168
Goldenrod, 168
Goldenseal, 3, 44, 50, 102, 107, **129**, 151, 168
Gotu kola, 126
Grapefruit seed extract, 85
Green tea, 44–45, 64, 85, 143
Grindelia, 147
Guggul, 116, 116–17, 144

H

Hawthorn, 45–46, 50, 115, 169
Henna, 26–27, 26–27
Hops, 120, 169
Horehound, 91
Horse chestnut, 160, 169
Horsetail, 136, 142, 169
Hyssop, 77

J

Jamaican dogwood, 169
Jasmine, 21
Juniper, 171

K

Kava kava, 46, 73, 73, 169
Korean ginseng, 43, 124, 126

L

Lady's-mantle, 46, 130
Lavender, 14, 18–19, 30, 46, 59, 62, 69, 83, 83, 110, **130**, 136, 141, 153–54, 154, 171
Lemon, 74, 171
Lemon balm, 14, 19–20, 46–47, 59, 61, 97, 110, 113, 115, 120, 131–32, **132**
Lemongrass, 171
Lemon thyme, 14
Licorice, 47, 47, 50, 66, 76, 90–91, 95, 111, 115, 131, 138, **138**, 156, 169

M

Marshmallow, 48, 151–52, 169
Meadowsweet, 137, 169
Medicago, 103
Milk thistle, 48, 130, 148
Milkweed, 35
Motherwort, 48, 50, 117, 119, 139
Mountain daisy, 3, 82, 135, 167
Mullein, 48–49, 82, 102, **141**
Myrrh, 93, 169

N

Nasturtium, 14
Nettle, 49, 51, 87, 108, 108, 134, 144, **146**, 169

O

Oak, 169
Oats, 86, 101, 138, 169
Oatmeal, 69, 86
Oatstraw, 51, 59, 97, 169
Olive oil, 93
Onion, 90, 115
Orange, 19, 131, 146, 171

P

Panax ginseng, 43, 124, 126
Papaya, 92–93

Parsley, 65–66, 70, 78, 82–83
Partridgeberry, 51
Passionflower, 50, 51, 59, 104
Peony, 103
Peppermint, 14, 16, 18, 20, 30, 51–52, 67, 79–80, 83,
        104, 106, 107, 109, 118, 131–33, **151**, 155,
        161, 171
Plantain, 50, **78–79**, 82
Psyllium, 112–13, 169

R

Red clover, 52
Red pepper. *See* Cayenne
Rhubarb, 50
Rose, 19, 21, 62, 146
Rose hip, 93
Rosemary, 14, 16, 18, 52–53, 100, 126, 126, 131, **153**,
        169, 172
Rue, 9, 169

S

Sage, 139, 169, 172
St. John's wort, 14, 30, 53, 86, 94, 96–97, 96, 101–2,
        144, 169
Sandalwood, 18, 74, 100, 136, 146, 158, 172
Sarsaparilla, 169
Sassafras, 170
Schisandra, 65–66, 144
Senna, 50
Shepherd's purse, 170
Siberian ginseng, 43, 66, 71, 105, 109, 119, 124,
        153
Skullcap, 50, 53, 59, 104, 128
Slippery elm, 11, 53–54, 92, 99, 102, 151, **157**,
        158–59

Soy extract, 145
Spearmint, 131–32, **160**
Stevia, 145
Stinging nettle. *See* Nettle
Strawberry, 141

T

Tang kuei, 103
Tea tree, 3, 77, 85, 158, 162–63, 172
Thuja, 162–63, 172
Thyme, 92, 172. *See also* Lemon thyme
Turmeric, 111, 170

U

Uva-ursi, 157

V

Valerian, 50, 54, 54–55, 73, 75, 103, 120–21,
        170
Vinegar, apple-cider, 95, 155, 159
Vitex, 2, 12, 36, 66, 103, 131, 139, 145–46, 168

W

White willow, 67, 110. *See also* Willow bark
Wild cherry, 77, 170
Willow bark, 106, 110, 134, 156, 170
Witch hazel, 3, 95, 112

Y

Yarrow, 2, 55, 106, 130, 146, **164**
Yellow dock, 50, 55, 148, 170
Ylang-ylang, 21, 146, 172

Subject Index

Boldface page references indicate illustrations. Underscored references indicate boxed text.

A

Abdominal cramps, 30
Acne, 68–69
Adaptogens, 71
Addiction
   caffeine, 84–85
   nicotine, 137–38
Age problems
   age spots, 69–70
   crow's-feet, 92–93
   herbs that fight, 42
   memory problems, 43, 125–26, 126
   menstrual flow, heavy, 129–30
   vaginal dryness, 158–59
   wrinkles, 92–93, 164–65, 165
Age spots, 69–70
AIDS, 85
Alcohol, 120
Alkaloids, 54
Allergies, 70–71
   chamomile, 36
   eczema and, 102
   essential oil, 18, 23, 60–61
   hay fever, 108–9, 108
   immune system and, 70
   insect bites and stings, 79
   poison plants, 146–47, 148, **149**
   sinusitis and, 150–51, 150
Allicin, 115
Alpha hydroxy acid, 70, 165
Alprazolam, 73
Altitude sickness, 71
American Association of Naturopathic Physicians,
   15
American Herbalists Guild, 15
American Holistic Medical Association, 15
Anemia, 71–72, 130
Anger, managing, 97
Antacids, 111
Antifungal soak, 77
Antihistamines, 70
Antioxidants, 53

Antiseptic herbs, 93
Anxiety, 61, 72–74, 73
Aphrodisiac, 21, 61, 125
Aromatherapy, 16, 17, 18
   equipment for, 17
   sexual attraction and, 21
   in treating
      depression, 97
      fatigue, 131
      low sexual desire, 125
      premenstrual syndrome, 146
      stress, 153
Arthritis, 34, 74–75, 74–75
Aspirin, 109–10
Asthma, 36, 45, 75–76, 76–77
Astringent herbs, 164
Athlete's foot, 76–77
Aveeno bath treatment, 86, 101

B

Bach Flower Remedies, 22
Back pain, 22–23
Bad breath, 77–79
Balms, herbal, 87, 153–54
Bath(s)
   Aveeno bath treatment and, 86, 101
   foot, 60, 77
   oils for, 97
   for relaxation, 60
   salts, 20, 60, 100
   sea salt, as alternative to, 19–20, 60
   sitz, 112
   in treating
      burns, 84
      colds, 19
      depression, 97
      genital itching, 86
      headaches, 110
      hemorrhoids, 112
      night sweats, 138–39
      stress, 153
      sunburn, 155

urinary tract infections, 158
vaginal itch, 159
Beans, 98, 106–7
Beer, 120
Berberine, 102, 107
Betulin, 161
Betulinic acid, 161
Bile, 69, 90, 119
Bites, insect, 44, 78–79, 79–80
Bitters, 51
Blackheads, 68
Blemishes, 68–69
Bloating, 128–29, 128, 146, 162–64
Blood pressure, 41. *See also* High blood
        pressure
Blood pressure screenings, 114
Blood-related problems, 71 –72, 130
Blues, 30, 33, 95–97, 96
Bone problems, 66, 141–42, 142–43
Botanical names of herbs, vs. common,
        12, 35
Bowel problems
    constipation, 90–91, 91
    diarrhea, 42, 98–99
Brands of herbal products, 13
Breast cancer, inflammatory, 73
Breastfeeding, 31, 80
Breast milk production, boosting, 80
Breast pain, 80–81
BreathAsure, 78
Breathing, calm, 73
Bronchitis, 81–82
Bruises, 82–83
Burns, 31, 83–84, 83

C

Caffeine
    addiction, 84–85
    benefits of, 105
    breast pain caused by, 81
    in chocolate, 84
    in coffee, 64, 84
    fatigue and, 105
    health problems caused by, 105
    menstruation and, 105
    in soda, 84
    in tea, 84
    wraps in drawing out toxin from, 19

Calcium
    menopause and, 66
    in nettle, 87
    in oatstraw, 51
    osteoporosis and, 66, 142, 142–43
    in red clover, 52
    in skullcap, 53
Calming herbs, 58–62, 59, 61
Candies, 22–23
Candles, 17
Canker sores, 85
Capsaicin, 75, 135
Capsules, 11
Carminatives, 107
Cervical changes, 85–86
Chapped lips, 86–87
Chloride, 99
Chlorophyll, 78
Chocolate, caffeine in, 84
Cholesterol levels, 41, 115–16, 116–17
Choosing herbs. *See* Herbs; Selecting herbal
        products
Chronic fatigue syndrome, 32–33
Cigarettes, 137–38, 165
Circulation, improving, 134
Cleansers, herbal, 101, 148
Cocktails, herbal, 61, 90, 118
Coffee, caffeine in, 64, 84, 105
Colas, caffeine in, 84
Colds
    incidence of, 87
    mysophobia and, 88–89
    treating
        baths, 19
        echinacea, 67, 88
        elderberry, 88
        garlic, 88
        ginger, 88–89
        nettle, 87
        soups, herbal, 45, 65
        teas, 87, 88–89
Collagen, 82
Colloidal oatmeal, 86, 147
Common names of herbs, vs. botanical, 12,
        35
Compress treatments, herbal
    for muscle strains and sprains, 135
    for puffy eyes, 149–50
    for sunburn, 154–55

Compress treatments, herbal *(continued)*
　for toothaches, 155–56
　for wound healing, 164
Concentration problems, <u>43</u>, 125–26, <u>126</u>
Conditioner, herbal hair, 100
Congestion, 16, 89–90
Constipation, 90–91, <u>91</u>
Cost of herbs, <u>44</u>
Coughs, 34, 91–92
Cough medicines, 20–21
Coumadin, 42
Cramps
　abdominal, 30
　menstrual, <u>103</u>, 128–29, <u>128</u>
　muscle, 134
Creams, herbal, 84, 86
Crow's-feet, 92–93
Culinary uses of herbs, <u>10</u>
Cuts, 31, 93–94
Cystic acne, 68

D

Dandruff, 94–95
Decoctions, <u>11</u>, 20
Dehydration, 99
Dental health, 78, 95, 107
Dental and mouth problems
　bad breath, 77–79
　canker sores, 85
　chapped lips, 86–87
　gum problems, 107–8
　plaque, 95, 107
　toothaches, 155–56
Depression, 95–97, <u>96</u>
Dermatitis, seborrheic, 94
Diabetes, 97–98
Diarrhea, 42, 98–99
Diazepam, 54, 71
Diet
　herbs in boosting nutrition in, <u>40</u>
　immune system and, 123–24
　importance of, 9
　overweight and, 142–43
　in treating
　　anemia, 72
　　breast pain, 81
　　diabetes, 98
　　high blood pressure, 114
Diffusers, <u>17</u>, 104

Digestion, 111, 119, 137
Digestive problems
　constipation, 90–91, <u>91</u>
　diarrhea, 42, 98–99
　gas, 106–7
　heartburn, 110–12, <u>112</u>
　indigestion, 16, <u>112</u>, 118–19, <u>118</u>
　nausea, 16, 42, 136–37, <u>137</u>
　ulcers, stomach, 36, 156–57
　upset stomach, 118–19, <u>118</u>
　vomiting, 136, 160–61
　water retention, 162–64
Dosages, herbal, 12–13, 67–68
Dramamine, 42, 133
Drugs. *See also specific names*
　depression caused by, 95
　herbs complementing, 68
　interactions with herbs, <u>50</u>
　side effects of, 67–68
Dry hair, 99–100
Dry skin, 100–101, <u>100</u>

E

Earaches, 101–2
Eczema, 102
EFAs, 39, 102
Emotional problems
　anger, 97
　anxiety, 61, 72–74, <u>73</u>
　depression, 95–97, <u>96</u>
　envy, <u>8–9</u>
　limbic system and, 73
　mood swings, 128
　mysophobia, <u>88–89</u>
　stress, 152–53
　　headaches and, 109, <u>109</u>
　　massage in relieving, <u>22</u>, 61–62
　　psoriasis and, 147
　　treating, <u>22</u>, 61–62, 152–53
Endometriosis, 102–4, <u>103</u>
Endorphins, 75
Energizing herbs, <u>32–33</u>, 63–66, <u>64</u>, <u>66</u>, 85
Envy, 8–9
Enzymes, 119
Esophageal reflux, 106
Essential fatty acids (EFAs), 39, 102
Essential oils, 18
　allergies to, 18, <u>23</u>, 60–61
　angelica, 73–74

eucalyptus, 81–82
with massage, 23
in onions, 90
peppermint, 79–80
recipe suggestions for, 18
safety issues, 68, 171–72
sexual attraction and, 21
shampoo and, 140
toxicity of, 18
in treating
dry and sun-damaged hair, 99–100
jet lag, 121
Estrogen. *See also* Hormonal imbalances
black cohosh and, 139
breast pain and, 80–81
hot flashes and, 117
menopause and, 126–27, 127, 139
perimenopause and, 144
Exercise, 9, 127, 153
Expiration dates on herbal products, 12
Extracts, 9–10
Eye problems, 98, 149–50

F

Facial masks, 101, 141, 165, 165
Facial peels, 69–70, 92–93, 165
Fatigue
caffeine and, 105
in midafternoon, 131–32
treating
aromatherapy, 131
basil, 105
dandelion, 132
ginseng, 105
peppermint, 67, 104, 131–32
teas, 65, 131–32
Fels Naptha soap, 147
Fen-phen, 144
Ferrous sulfate, 72
Fever, 105–6
Fiber, 90, 98, 112–13
First-aid herb kit, 3
Flatulence, 106–7
Flower essences, 21–22
Flu, 45, 65, 85–89, 87
Fluoride, 95
Footbaths, herbal, 60, 77. *See also* Baths
Foot problems, 76–77
Fungus, 76–77, 94

G

Gas, 106–7
Genital warts, 85–86
Germs, fear of, 88–89
Ginger ale, 106, 118
Gingerols, 118
Gingivitis, 107–8
Ginkgolides, 70
Glycyrrhizin, 47, 76, 95
Gum problems, 107–8

H

Hair coloring, 26–27, 26–27
Hair problems
dandruff, 94–95
dry hair, 99–100
oily hair, 139–40, 140
rinses in treating, 94–95
sun-damaged hair, 99–100
Hair therapies, 26–27, 26–27
Halitosis, 77–79
Hay fever, 108–9, 108. *See also* Allergies
HDL, 115–16
Headaches
causes of, 109, 109
massage and, 22–23
migraines, 132
stress and, 109, 109
tension, 22–23, 132
treating
aspirin, 109–10
baths, 110
cramp bark, 110
feverfew, 41, 110
ginkgo, 71
teas, 110
white willow, 67
Health problems. *See specific types*
Heartburn, 110–12, 112. *See also* Indigestion
Heart disease risk, garlic in reducing, 116
Helenalin, 82
Helicobacter pylori, 157
Hemoglobin, 71–72
Hemorrhoids, 16, 112–13
Henna paste, 26–27, 26–27
Herbs, 6, 7–9. *See also* Selecting herbal products
antiseptic, 93
astringent, 164

Herbs *(continued)*
  availability of, 67–68
  botanical names of, 12, <u>35</u>
  brands of, 13
  calming, 58–62, <u>59</u>, <u>61</u>
  common names of, 12, <u>35</u>
  cost of, <u>44</u>
  culinary uses of, <u>10</u>
  dosages of, 12–13, 67–68
  drug interactions and, <u>50</u>
  energizing, <u>32–33</u>, 63–66, <u>64</u>, <u>66</u>, 85
  in first-aid kit, <u>3</u>
  growing, on windowsill, <u>14</u>
  historical perspective of, 2, <u>31</u>
  important, 30–55
    aloe, 31–32, <u>31</u>
    angelica, 32
    astragalus, 32–33, <u>32–33</u>
    basil, 33
    bearberry, 33–34
    black cohosh, 34
    black haw, 34
    blue cohosh, 34
    burdock, 34–35
    calendula, 35
    chamomile, 35–36
    chasteberry, 36
    comfrey, 36
    cramp bark, 36–37
    dandelion, 37, <u>37</u>
    dong quai, 38
    echinacea, 38
    eucalyptus, 39
    evening primrose, <u>38–39</u>, 39–40
    fennel, 40
    feverfew, 40–41
    garlic, <u>40</u>, 41–42, <u>41</u>
    ginger, 42
    ginkgo, 42, <u>43</u>
    ginseng, 43
    goldenseal, 44
    green tea, 44–45
    hawthorn, 45–46
    kava kava, 46
    lady's-mantle, 46
    lavender, 46
    lemon balm, 46–47
    licorice, 47, <u>47</u>
    marshmallow, 48
    milk thistle, 48
    motherwort, 48
    mullein, 48–49
    nettle, 49, 51
    oatstraw, 51
    partridgeberry, 51
    peppermint, 51–52
    red clover, 52
    rosemary, 52–53
    St. John's wort, 53
    skullcap, 53
    slippery elm, 53–54
    valerian, 54, <u>54–55</u>
    yarrow, 55
    yellow dock, 55
  limitations of, 9
  nutrition with, <u>40</u>
  in office mini-kit, <u>52</u>
  organic, 13
  popularity of, renewed, 2–3, <u>31</u>
    reasons for, 4–6
  pregnancy and, 68
  safety issues, 13–15, 31, 68, 167–70
  serenity, 58–62, <u>59</u>, <u>61</u>
  side effects of, 8, 31, 68
  storing, 15
  supplements and, vitamin and mineral, <u>66</u>
  terminology of, 9–11, <u>11</u>
  versatility of, 8–9
  women and use of, 3–4
Herbalist, selecting, <u>4–5</u>
Herpes simplex, 35, 113–14
High blood pressure, 114–15, <u>114–15</u>
High cholesterol, 115–16, <u>116–17</u>
High-density lipoprotein (HDL), 115–16
Histamines, 70, 108
Hoarseness, 122
Hormonal imbalances
  energy levels and, 63
  liver and, 130
  menopause and, 126–27, <u>127</u>
  supplements and, vitamin and mineral, <u>66</u>
  treating
    chasteberry, <u>66</u>
    tonic, herbal, 81, 130
Hormone-replacement therapy (HRT), 127, <u>143</u>
Hot flashes, 49, <u>66</u>, 116–17, 128, <u>139</u>
HPV, 85–86, 161–62
HRT, 127, <u>143</u>

Human papillomavirus (HPV), 85–86, 161–62
Hydrastine, 107
Hydrotherapy. *See* Baths
Hypericin, 53, 97
Hypertension, 114–15, <u>114–15</u>

I

Ice treatments, 82–83, 134–35
Immune system
  allergies and, 70
  boosting
    astragalus, 32, <u>40</u>
    comfrey, 36
    echinacea, 80, 102, <u>124</u>
    garlic, 86, 125
    St. John's wort, 86
    soup, herbal, <u>45</u>
  diet and, 123–24
  massage and, <u>22</u>
  weak, 123–25, <u>124</u>
Indigestion, 16, <u>112</u>, 118–19, <u>118</u>. *See also* Heartburn
Indole, 95
Infections
  bladder, 33
  energy levels and, 63
  fungal, 94
  kidney, <u>158–59</u>
  sinusitis, 150–51, <u>150</u>
  treating
    comfrey, 36
    sandalwood, 16
    slippery elm, 54
  urinary tract, 33, 157–58, <u>158–59</u>
  yeast, 94
Infertility, <u>105</u>, 119
Inflammation. *See* Infections
Infusions, <u>11</u>, 20
Ingredients in herbal products, 13
Insect bites and stings, 44, <u>78–79</u>, 79–80
Insomnia
  alcohol and, <u>120</u>
  schisandra in rebounding from, 65
  treating
    lemon balm, 120
    sleep pillow, herbal, <u>122–23</u>
    teas, <u>61</u>, 120–21, <u>120</u>
    valerian, <u>54–55</u>, 120–21
Insulin, 97–98

Interferon, 88
Iron, 53, 72, <u>87</u>
Iron-deficiency anemia, 72, 130
Isoflavones, 127

J

Jet lag, 121
Jewelweed, **148**, <u>148</u>
Joint problems, 74–75, <u>74–75</u>
Juice, herbal, 123

K

Kavalactones, 73
Kidney infection, <u>158–59</u>

L

Labels, reading herbal, 11–13
Lactation, promoting, 80
Lactose, 106
Lactose intolerance, 106
Lamp rings, <u>17</u>
Laryngitis, 122
Lawsone, <u>148</u>
LDL, 115–16
Leg problems
  muscle cramps, 134
  varicose veins, 159–60
Length of herbal use, 15
Licorice candy, <u>47</u>
Limbic system, 73
Lips, chapped, 86–87
Liver, protecting, 130
Liver spots, 69–70
Low-density lipoprotein (LDL), 115–16
Low immunity, 123–25, <u>124</u>
Low sexual desire, 125
Lozenges, herbal, 22–23, 92
Lung ailments, 36. *See also* Respiratory problems

M

Magnesium, 52–53, 87
Magnesium citrate, <u>66</u>
Masks, facial, 101, 141, 165, <u>165</u>
Massage, <u>22–23</u>, 134–36
  oils, <u>22</u>, 23–24, 62

Medical conditions. *See specific types*
Melanin, 69, 86
Memory problems, <u>43</u>, 125–26, <u>126</u>
Menopause
   calcium and, <u>66</u>
   estrogen and, 126–27, <u>127</u>, <u>139</u>
   hormonal imbalances and, 126–27, <u>127</u>
   hot flashes and, <u>49</u>, <u>66</u>, 116–17, 128, <u>139</u>
   night sweats and, 138–39, <u>139</u>
   treating symptoms of
      black cohosh, <u>66</u>, <u>127</u>, <u>139</u>
      chasteberry, <u>139</u>
      hormone-replacement therapy, 127
      tonic, herbal, <u>49</u>
Menstruation
   caffeine and, <u>105</u>
   constipation and, 90
   cramps during, <u>103</u>, 128–29, <u>128</u>
   heavy flow, 129–30
   irregularity, 130–31
Metabolism, 143
Midafternoon slump, 131–32
Migraines, 132
Minerals. *See specific names*
Mineral supplements, <u>66</u>
Miracle claims, avoiding, 13
Mists, herbal, <u>17</u>
Moisturizers, 69, 92, 101, 102
Mood swings, 128
Motion sickness, 42, 132–34, <u>133</u>
Mouth problems. *See* Dental and mouth
      problems
Mouth ulcers, 85
Mouthwashes, 78, 95
Mucilage, 48, 92, 99, 102
Muscle problems
   aches, 36–37, 88–89
   cramps, 134
   sprains, 134–36, <u>135</u>
   strains, 134–36, <u>135</u>
Mysophobia, <u>88–89</u>

N

Nail problems, 136
Nardil, 42
Nasal problems
   congestion, 16, 89–90
   postnasal drip, chronic, <u>133</u>

sinusitis, 150–51, <u>150</u>
   vomiting and, 136
National Commission for Certification for
      Acupuncture and Oriental Medicine, 15
Nausea treatments
   dandelion, 137
   ginger, 42, 88–89, 137
   meadowsweet, 137
   peppermint, 16
   tonic, herbal, <u>137</u>
Nervines, 46
Nicotine, <u>19</u>
Nicotine withdrawal, 137–38
Night sweats, 138–39, <u>139</u>
Nipples, sore, 80
Non-insulin-dependent diabetes, 97–98
Nonsteroidal anti-inflammatory medications, 42
Nutrition with herbs, boosting, <u>40</u>

O

Oatmeal, 86, 147
Odors. *See* Aromatherapy
Office mini-kit of herbs, <u>52</u>
Oily hair, 139–40, <u>140</u>
Oily skin, 141
Organic herbs, 13
Osteoarthritis, 74. *See also* Arthritis
Osteoporosis, <u>66</u>, 141–42, <u>142–43</u>
Overweight, 142–44, <u>145</u>
Oxygen, 71–72

P

Pain. *See also* Headaches
   arthritis, 34, 74–75, <u>74–75</u>
   back, <u>22–23</u>
   breast, 80–81
   bruises, 82–83
   burns, 83–84, <u>83</u>
   cayenne and, 75, <u>135</u>
   cramps
      abdominal, 30
      menstrual, 34, <u>103</u>, 128–29, <u>128</u>
      muscle, 134
   from cuts and scrapes, 94
   ear, 101–2
   endometriosis, 102–4, <u>103</u>
   hemorrhoidal, 16, 112–13

insect bites and stings, <u>78–79</u>, 79–80
migraines, 132
muscle, 36–37, 88–89
St. John's wort and, 94
sprains, muscle, 134–36, <u>135</u>
strains, muscle, 134–36, <u>135</u>
sunburn, 154–55, <u>154</u>
tooth, 155–56
ulcer, 156–57
varicose vein, 159–60
Pap test, 86
Parnate, 42
Pastes, herbal, 102
Peels, facial, 69–70, 92–93, 165
Penicillin, discovery of, 4
Perimenopause, 144–45
Periodontitis, 107
Peristalsis, 118
Phenelzine sulfate, 42
Phlegm, 81, 91, 123
Physical activity, 9, 127, 153
Phytoestrogens, <u>143</u>
Pimples, 68–69
Pituitary gland, 131
Plaque, dental, 95, 107
PMS, 36, <u>66</u>, <u>105</u>, 146
Poison ivy, 146–47, <u>148</u>, **149**
Poison oak, 146–47, <u>148</u>, **149**
Poison plants, 146–47, **148**, <u>149</u>
Poison sumac, 146–47, <u>148</u>, **149**
Popsicle, herbal, 61
Postnasal drip, chronic, <u>133</u>
Potassium, 52–53, <u>87</u>, 99
Potpourri, 27
Poultices, 11, 80, 82, 135
Powders, 11
Pregnancy
    constipation during, <u>91</u>
    gum problems and, 107
    herbs and, 68
    sebum production and, 139–40
Premenstrual syndrome (PMS), 36, <u>66</u>, <u>105</u>, 146
Prescription medications. *See also specific names*
    depression caused by, 95
    herbs complementing, 68
    interactions with herbs, <u>50</u>
    side effects of, 67–68
Progesterone, 126, 129, 144. *See also* Hormonal
        imbalances

Properdin, 88
Proteins, 88, 106
Prozac, <u>96</u>
Psoriasis, <u>38–39</u>, 147–48
Puffy eyes, 149–50

Q

Quercetin, 70–71, 98
Quiz, about herbs, <u>6</u>

R

Red blood cells, 71–72
Relaxation, baths for, 60
Reproductive problems
    endometriosis, 102–4, <u>103</u>
    infertility, <u>105</u>, 119
    low sexual desire, 125
    menstrual cramps, <u>103</u>, 128–29, <u>128</u>
    menstrual flow, heavy, 129–30
    menstrual irregularity, 130–31
    premenstrual syndrome, 36, <u>66</u>, <u>105</u>, 146
    vaginal dryness, 158–59
    vaginal itch, 159
Respiratory problems. *See also* Allergies
    asthma, 36, 45, 75–76, <u>76–77</u>
    bronchitis, 81–82
    congestion, 16, 89–90
    coughs, 34, 91–92
    hay fever, 108–9, <u>108</u>
Rheumatoid arthritis, 74. *See also* Arthritis
Rinses, herbal, 85, 94–95, 140, 151
Rubs, herbal, 74, 82, 135, 155

S

Sachet, making, 27
Safety issues
    essential oils, 68, 171–72
    herbs and herbal products, 13–15, 31, 68,
        167–70
    seals on herbal products, 12
Salad, dandelion, 72
Salicin, 106
Salicylates, 75
Salicylic acid, 110
Salt, 99
Salts, bath, 20, 60, <u>100</u>

Salves, herbal, 84, 86
Sanguinarine, 95
Scalds, 31, 83–84, 83
Scents. *See* Aromatherapy
Schizandrin, 144
Scrapes, 31, 93–94
Scrubs, cleansing, 24–25, 69
Sea salt, 20, 60
Sea sickness, 132–34, 133
Seborrheic dermatitis, 94
Sebum, 68, 139–40
Selecting herbal products
  brands and, 13
  dosages and, 12–13
  experts and, relying on, 14–15
  expiration dates and, 12
  herbalist and, 4–5
  ingredients in products and, 13
  labels and, reading, 11–13
  length of product use and, 15
  miracle claims and, avoiding, 13
  organic products and, 13
  safety issues and, 13–15
  shopping skills needed for, 7
  single-herb products and, 13
  terminology and, learning, 9–11, 11
  understanding herbs and, 7–9
Serenity herbs, 58–62, 59, 61
Sexual attraction, essential oils and, 21
Sexual desire, low, 125
Shampoo, herbal, 140, 140
Shogaols, 118
Side effects
  of drugs, 68
  of herbs, 8, 31, 68
Silica, 136
Silicic acid, 51
Silicon, 142
Silymarin, 48, 130
Single-herb products, 13
Sinusitis, 150–51, 150
Sitz baths, 112
Skin care, 24–26, 30, 68–69, 99–100
Skin problems
  acne, 68–69
  age spots, 69–70
  athlete's foot, 76–77
  bruises, 82–83
  burns, 31, 83–84, 83

  chapped lips, 86–87
  crow's-feet, 92–93
  cuts, 31, 93–94
  dandruff, 94–95
  dermatitis, seborrheic, 94
  dry skin, 100–101, 100
  eczema, 102
  insect bites and stings, 44, 78–79, 79–80
  oily skin, 141
  poison plants and, 146–47, **148–49**, 149
  psoriasis, 38–39, 147–48
  scalds, 31, 83–84, 83
  scrapes, 31, 93–94
  stretch marks, 153–54
  sunburn, 154–55, 154
  warts, 161–62, 162–63
  wrinkles, 92–93, 164–65, 165
Sleeping problems. *See also* Insomnia
  menopause and, 66
  night sweats, 138–39, 139
  treating
    schisandra, 65
    sleep pillow, herbal, 121, 122–23
Sleep pillow, herbal, 121, 122–23
Smoking, quitting, 137–38, 165
Soaks, herbal, 60, 77, 161. *See also* Baths
Sodas
  caffeine in, 84
  cavities and, 95
Sodium, 99
Soluble fiber, 98
Sorbitol, 106
Sore throats, 16, 151–52, 152
Soups, herbal, 45, 65–66, 71, 98
Soy milk, 143
SPF, 154
Sprains, muscle, 134–36, 135
Sprays, herbal, 20, 62, 154
Steams, herbal, 89, 122–23, 141, 151
Stings, insect, 44, 78–79, 79–80
Stomach acid, 111
Stomach ulcers, 36, 156–57
Stomach upsets, 118–19, 118. *See also* Nausea
    treatments
Storing herbs, 15
Strains, muscle, 134–36, 135
Stress, 152–53
  aromatherapy in relieving, 153
  headaches and, 109, 109

massage in relieving, <u>22</u>, 61–62
psoriasis and, 147
treating, <u>22</u>, 61–62, 152–53
Stretch marks, 153–54
Stuffy nose, 89–90
Substance P, <u>135</u>
Sugar levels, 98
Sulfur, 106
Sunburn, 154–55, <u>154</u>
Sun-damaged hair, 99–100
Sun protection factor (SPF), 154
Sunscreen, 69, 92, 154
Supplements, vitamin and mineral, <u>40</u>, <u>66</u>, 72,
    <u>143</u>

T

Tannins, 46, 51, 154–55
Tea(s), 10
   for baths, 60
   burdock, 69, 94, 113–14
   caffeine in, 84
   calendula, 80
   chamomile, 107, 111–12, 121, 149–50
   corn silk, 163
   dandelion, 150, 161
   dill, <u>112</u>
   echinacea, 102, 113–14
   fennel, 80, 149
   fluoride in, 95
   ginger, 74, 88–89, 137
   ginger ale, 106, <u>118</u>
   green, 85, 143
   hair rinse, 26
   horsetail, 142
   iron-rich, 72
   lactation-promoting, 80
   licorice-prune, 90–91
   marshmallow, 151–52
   meadowseet, 137
   motherwort, 139
   mullein, 82
   nettle, <u>87</u>, 108
   peppermint, 107, 118, 133–34, 161
   plantain, 82
   for relaxation, 60
   sage, 139
   tannic acid in, 154
   thyme, 92

in treating
   arthritis, 75
   bad breath, 79
   colds, <u>87</u>, 88–89
   constipation, 90–91
   coughs, 20–21, 92
   depression, 97
   diabetes, 98
   diarrhea, 99
   earache, 102
   endometriosis, 103–4
   fatigue, 65, 131–32
   fever, 106
   gas, 106
   gum problems, 107
   hay fever, 108
   headaches, 110
   heartburn, 111–12, <u>112</u>
   herpes, 113–14
   indigestion, <u>112</u>, 118
   infertility, 119
   insomnia, <u>61</u>, 120–21, <u>120</u>
   jet lag, 121
   low sexual desire, 125
   menstrual cramps, 129
   menstrual irregularity, 131
   motion sickness, 133–34
   muscle aches, 88–89
   nausea, 88–89, 137
   nicotine withdrawal, 138
   night sweats, 139
   osteoporosis, 142
   overweight, 143
   puffy eyes, 149–50
   sore throats, 151–52, <u>152</u>
   ulcers, 156–57
   vomiting, 161
   water retention, 163–64
Tension headaches, <u>22–23</u>, 132
Tension. *See* Stress
Terminology, herbal, 9–11, <u>11</u>
Terpenes, 42–43
Therapies, herbal. *See also* Aromatherapy
   baths, 18–20
   candies, 22–23
   cough medicines, 20–21
   flower essences, 21–22
   for hair, 26–27, <u>26–27</u>
   lozenges, 22 –23, 92

Therapies *(continued)*
    massage, <u>22–23</u>
        oils, <u>22</u>, 23–24
    potpourri, 27
    for skin, 24–26
    wraps, <u>19</u>
Throat problems
    laryngitis, 122
    sore throat, 16, 151–52, <u>152</u>
Tinctures, 9–10
Toners, skin, 24–125
Tonics, herbal
    for breast pain, 81
    energy-boosting, 85
    for liver production, 130
    for menopausal symptoms, <u>49</u>
    for nausea, <u>137</u>
    for urinary tract infections, 157
Toothaches, 155–56
Toothpaste, herbal, 107, <u>155</u>
Topical beauty therapies, 24–26, 30
Toxins, 63, 99, 148
Tranquilizers, 54, 73
Tranylcypromine, 42
Travel-related problems
    altitude sickness, 71
    jet lag, 121
    motion sickness, 42, 132–34, <u>133</u>
Type I diabetes, 97
Type II diabetes, 97–98

U

Ulcers
    mouth, 85
    stomach, 36, 156–57
Upset stomach, 118–19, <u>118</u>. *See also* Nausea
    treatments
Urinary tract infection (UTI), 33, 157–58,
    <u>158–59</u>
Urushiol, 147
UTI, 33, 157–58, <u>158–59</u>

V

Vaginal creams, herbal, 86, 158–59
Vaginal dryness, 158–59

Vaginal itch, 159
Valium, 54, 73
Vapors, herbal, 81–82
Varicose veins, 159–60
Vegetables, 72
Viadent, 95
Viruses, <u>45</u>, 64, 85–89, <u>87</u>
Vitamin A, <u>84</u>
Vitamin B_6, <u>66</u>, 146
Vitamin B_{12}, 38
Vitamin C, 52, 84, <u>87</u>, 154
Vitamin D, 142
Vitamin E, 38, 84, 136, 142, 154, 158–59
Vitamin supplements, <u>40</u>, <u>66</u>
Vomiting, 136, 160–61

W

Wafarin, 42
Warts
    genital, 85–86
    topical skin, 161–62, <u>162–63</u>
Waste elimination, improved, 68–69, 74–75
Water, herbal-scented, <u>20</u>
Water intake, 100–101, 112, 167
Water jet, dental, 107
Water Pik, 107
Water retention, 162–64
Weight problems, 142–44, <u>145</u>
Wheezing, 70, 108
Whiteheads, 68
Windowsill herbs, <u>14</u>
Wound healing, 84, 164
Wraps, herbal, <u>19</u>
Wrinkles, 92–93, 164–65, <u>165</u>

X

Xanax, 73

Y

Yeast infections, 94

Z

Zinc, 84, <u>87</u>, 88–89, 154